Common Neuro-Ophthalmic Pitfalls

Case-Based Teaching

Valerie A. Purvin

Aki Kawasaki

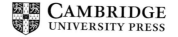

CAMBRIDGE
UNIVERSITY PRESS

CAMBRIDGE UNIVERSITY PRESS

Cambridge, New York, Melbourne, Madrid, Cape Town, Singapore, São Paulo, Delhi

Cambridge University Press
The Edinburgh Building, Cambridge CB2 8RU, UK

Published in the United States of America by Cambridge University Press, New York

www.cambridge.org
Information on this title: www.cambridge.org/9780521713269

First published 2009

Printed in the United Kingdom at the University Press, Cambridge

A catalog record for this publication is available from the British Library

Library of Congress Cataloging in Publication data
Purvin, Valerie A., 1948–
Common neuro-ophthalmologic pitfalls / by Valerie A. Purvin and Aki Kawasaki.
 p. ; cm.
Includes bibliographical references and index.
ISBN 978-0-521-71326-9
1. Neuroophthalmology – Case studies. I. Kawasaki, Aki. II. Title.
[DNLM: 1. Eye Diseases – diagnosis – Case Reports. 2. Eye Diseases – therapy –
Case Reports. 3. Diagnostic Errors – prevention & control – Case Reports.
4. Nervous System Diseases – diagnosis – Case Reports. 5. Nervous System
Diseases – therapy – Case Reports. WW 140 P986c 2009]
RE725.P87 2009
617.7′32 – dc22   2008038180

ISBN 978-0-521-71326-9 paperback

Contents

Foreword

If you have already bought this book, you made the right choice. If you are just browsing through it and trying to decide whether to buy it, you must be tempted. Go ahead – you will not be disappointed.

This is the work of two gifted clinicians. With deep credentials in academic neuro-ophthalmology and frequent performances on the lecture circuit, they are highly respected in their field. What makes them especially distinctive is that they not only understand neuro-ophthalmic disease, they catch its finest nuances and they know how to share them – and teach them.

If you think you need a straight-up textbook to learn this material, think again. Reading a textbook might be like using a guidebook to go through an art museum. Reading this book is like having a personal guide who is both erudite and passionate. It is much more fun.

The subject matter is all cases – real cases that the authors have grappled with. Each illustrates a critical problem in neuro-ophthalmic diagnosis or management. Because we learn best when we make mistakes, the authors have selected cases in which someone stumbled.

The cases are presented as mystery stories. Whether you are a neuro-ophthalmic novice or a sophisticate, an ophthalmologist or a neurologist, a physician in training or a physician in practice, you will enjoy matching your wits against these gurus!

Jonathan D. Trobe, MD
University of Michigan

Preface

This book is a case-based teaching tool, meant to bridge the gap between textbook information and the everyday experience of the clinician "in the trenches". Our intended audience includes medical students, residents and practitioners in the fields of neurology, ophthalmology, neurosurgery and neuroradiology as well as our colleagues specializing in neuro-ophthalmology.

The level of information provided in these case discussions assumes that the reader has some degree of familiarity with basic anatomic pathways and with the pathophysiology of common neuro-ophthalmic disorders. There are a number of excellent textbooks that cover this kind of information and the reader is directed to these sources for review and expansion of this information as needed. The case discussions do include a brief review of key points regarding neuroanatomy and physiology when relevant, highlighting those with direct clinical correlation.

The choice of cases is to some extent arbitrary. The book is not meant to be inclusive but rather to illustrate diagnostic principles, trying to focus on those that are a frequent source of confusion or discomfort, especially to the non-ophthalmologist. In each case we try to highlight the specific aspect of the clinical presentation that points to the correct diagnosis, furnished as the "tip" at the end of the case discussion.

Because the text is not organized anatomically or by disease process, certain disorders appear in more than one location. This occurs because of the diverse clinical manifestations of certain conditions. For example, the features of an Adie's pupil when acute (unilateral dilated pupil) are distinct from those when the disorder is chronic (bilateral small poorly reactive pupils). Similarly, the clinical presentations of Leber's hereditary optic neuropathy and dominant optic atrophy are quite different even though both are forms of hereditary optic nerve disease. These different sections are meant to be complementary. Care has been taken to avoid redundancy or repetition and in each case the reader is directed to the location of the additional information. Each case can stand alone as a complete story, however, and so the book can be read in any order. We hope this format is user-friendly and would like to think that our readers will find the book "a fun read".

Although a variety of disorders and different kinds of "pitfalls" are covered, there is a clear recurring theme in these cases, namely the importance of information derived from the history and the physical examination in the diagnosis of neuro-ophthalmic disease. Advances in modern neuroimaging sometimes create the impression that such "old-fashioned" clinical skills are no longer necessary, that they are an anachronism. These cases illustrate the way in which such clinical skill complements and informs the data that we obtain from ancillary testing.

Acknowledgements

We would like to thank a number of people for their assistance with this book. We are particularly grateful to Yann Leuba for his expert assistance with the figures and to Shelley Wood for many technical aspects of the project. We greatly appreciate the input of Benjamin Kuzma on many aspects of neuro-imaging. Many thanks to our colleagues Francois-Xavier Borruat, Daryel Ellis, Richard Burgett and John Minturn for their very helpful suggestions on selected chapters. Our special thanks go to Jonathan Trobe for his reading of the entire manuscript and offering such nuanced and insightful comments and criticism. Finally, we appreciate the longtime support of Donald Wilson and the Midwest Eye Foundation.

When ocular disease is mistaken for neurologic disease

Some common visual symptoms, such as blurring, double vision and flashing lights, can be produced by disorders of either the eye or the brain. Sorting out ocular disease early in the course of the evaluation is important for avoiding unnecessary and often expensive investigation, establishing a definitive diagnosis and initiating appropriate treatment. While the non-ophthalmologists cannot be expected to have the tools and refined examination skills of the ophthalmologist, there are some specific clinical findings that can help in distinguishing between eye and brain disease.

In many cases, a detailed description of the visual symptom effectively localizes the disease process. For example, visual loss due to aberration of the ocular media (e.g. cataract or corneal disease) is usually described as "blurring", while the visual loss of optic nerve dysfunction is more often experienced as "dimming" or "darkening", often with decreased color saturation (Figure 1.1). In contrast to patients with disorders of the media, those with retinal or optic nerve disease often report missing "pieces" or areas of vision. Alteration of object shape or size (metamorphopsia, micropsia or macropsia) usually indicates retinal disease and is never caused by optic neuropathy. Prominent degradation of vision in dim or bright light is also characteristic of retinal disease. Familiarity with such distinctive features of the history is particularly important for the clinician, particularly the non-ophthalmologist, because in such cases sophisticated eye examination techniques are not necessary to know that the disease process is an ocular one.

A   B   C

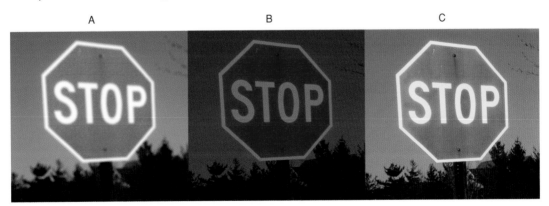

Figure 1.1 Comparison of subjective visual abnormality in ocular vs. neurologic disease. (A) Disorders of the ocular media usually produce *blurring* of images, with loss of sharp edges. (B) Patients with optic neuropathies often describe *dimming* of images and (C) color desaturation. (Figure courtesy of Stuart Alfred.)

In some instances, the history is non-specific, and localization rests on specific examination findings and techniques. The photostress test and Amsler grid are two such examples. The *photostress test* measures the time it takes to recover central visual function, e.g. acuity following exposure to a bright light, and is very useful for distinguishing maculopathy from optic neuropathy. Recovery times are prolonged in a variety of macular disorders but are normal in optic neuropathies. *Amsler grid testing* is an objective way to assess alteration of object shape and size, a characteristic of macular disease (see Chapter 8, Sudden difficulty reading the paper). In yet other cases, a particular aspect of the eye examination that requires some experience and expertise, such as inspection of the drainage angle (gonioscopy) or visualization of the peripheral retina (scleral depression), provides the key to the correct diagnosis. While such examination techniques are beyond the purview of the non-ophthalmologist, it is crucial to know when the patient should be referred for such examination. The section that follows looks at some examples of cases in which the findings that indicate ocular disease were either subtle, absent or misinterpreted.

Double images

Case: A 60-year-old seamstress sought medical attention because of a three-month history of intermittent diplopia that was most noticeable in the evening, particularly when driving. She found she could relieve her diplopia by closing her right eye. She had no head or eye pain and no recent systemic symptoms. On examination, ocular alignment was normal and eye movements in all directions were full. Refixation saccades were brisk and accurate and there was no ptosis or lid fatigability. Thyroid function tests and a magnetic resonance imaging (MRI) scan of brain and orbits were normal. Her history of intermittent diplopia that was worse at night suggested the possibility of myasthenia, and further work-up was initiated accordingly. Acetylcholine receptor antibodies were negative, electromyography (EMG) with repetitive stimulation showed no decrement, and a trial of Mestinon (pyridostigmine bromide) did not bring symptomatic relief.

The patient returned several months later reporting that her diplopia had now become constant. Her examination was unchanged.

What important piece of historical information is still missing in this case?

The work-up so far has assumed this patient's diplopia was binocular but in fact all that we know is that it was relieved by closing her *right* eye. In order to establish that this is not monocular double vision we also need to know what happens when she closes the left eye. With her left eye closed, viewing just with the right, she described persistence of her double images.

What maneuver might be helpful for confirming our suspicion that this patient's double vision is ocular in nature?

The *pinhole test* is useful when aberration of the ocular media or refractive error is the basis of visual disturbance, including both blurring and doubling of vision (Figure 1.2). By allowing only a small bundle of incoming light rays to enter the eye, only those that are parallel to the visual axis reach the retina. The amount of light scatter onto the retina, and thus image degradation, is therefore greatly reduced. Patients who complain of blur, halos, shadowy margins and monocular double vision will note improved image clarity or even complete resolution of symptoms when viewing through a pinhole.

This patient's diplopia was indeed relieved by pinhole. Slit-lamp examination demonstrated a developing cataract in the right eye and was otherwise normal. In retrospect, her history had been misleading. Because she reported resolution of diplopia upon covering her right eye, it was thought that she had binocular diplopia, but in reality, her diplopia was present only in the right eye. Further questioning would have revealed that diplopia

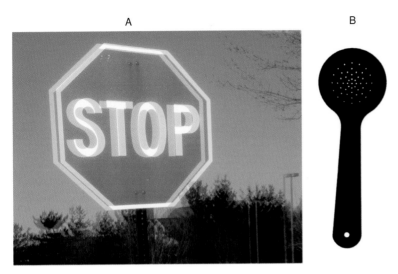

Figure 1.2 Monocular diplopia due to aberration of the ocular media. (A) Double image is present with just one eye viewing. Note the second image has a faded appearance, sometimes termed a "ghost" image. (B) A pinhole occluder relieves diplopia due to ocular aberration.

resolved only with covering the right eye and not the left eye, clearly indicating monocular diplopia.

Her diplopia resolved completely after cataract extraction.

Discussion: For practical purposes, monocular diplopia or polyopia (multiple images present with just one eye viewing) is due to an aberration of the ocular media, not neurologic disease. Common causes include uncorrected refractive errors, corneal disease, cataract and macular distortion. Monocular diplopia is often less noticeable when outdoors or in a brightly lit room, because the resulting pupillary constriction induces a pinhole-like effect. Symptoms are often more noticeable in dim illumination and at nighttime, especially when driving.

Corneal surface disease related to dry eyes is an important cause of monocular diplopia. Drying of the corneal surface is a common age-related change and also occurs in a variety of other settings, including after blepharoplasty (due to increased lid height and tear evaporation), with the use of anticholinergic or antihistaminic agents (decreased tear production), contact lens wear (surface irritation),

and low-humidity environments. Patients with thyroid eye disease are particularly prone to dry eyes because of lid retraction and lacrimal gland infiltration. Symptoms include burning, foreign-body sensation, blur, photosensitivity, halos around lights, and diplopia. Paradoxically, excessive watering is also a common symptom of dry eyes, caused by increased reflex tearing which produces thin, watery tears that are less effective than normal tear secretion. Symptoms related to dry eyes are often intermittent, typically made worse by prolonged viewing (e.g. reading or computer use) during which the cornea dries out from decreased blinking. Patients with parkinsonian syndromes are also prone to this condition, as a consequence of their decreased blink rate.

The one exception to the dictum that monocular diplopia indicates ocular disease is a rare neurologic condition called *cerebral polyopia*. Cerebral polyopia is a visual illusion, usually due to parietal lobe dysfunction, in which objects are seen as multiple (two or more) in each eye. In most cases, cerebral polyopia is associated with other forms of higher cortical visual disturbance, such as abnormal persistence of images and spatial distortion.

Cerebral polyopia can be distinguished from monocular polyopia due to disorders of the ocular media by the following: (1) cerebral polyopia is always present in both eyes, (2) cerebral polyopia is *not* relieved by pinhole, and (3) cerebral polyopia is usually associated with homonymous visual field defects.

Before embarking on a neurologic evaluation for diplopia, it is important to verify that diplopia is truly binocular. If it is, the patient should note resolution of diplopia when *either* eye is covered.

Diagnosis: Monocular diplopia due to cataract

Tip: Diplopia that is present with one eye viewing and relieved by pinhole is not due to neurologic disease.

Headache and bilateral disc edema

Case: A 37-year-old schoolbus driver noted rapidly progressive visual blur in both eyes. He did not have eye pain but reported intense daily headaches which had started three months previously. He was unaware of any medical problems and was taking no medications. Examination revealed visual acuity of 20/40 in each eye and bilateral optic disc edema (Figure 1.3A). Visual field testing showed central depression and paracentral scotomas in both eyes (Figure 1.3B). There was no alteration of sensorium and no focal neurologic deficits. A brain tumor was suspected and he was sent as an emergency for an MRI, which was normal. He was scheduled for a lumbar puncture, but while the procedure was pending a bedside test was performed, leading to a definitive diagnosis.

What test was done and what was the diagnosis?

His blood pressure was checked and found to be markedly elevated at 240/170. An ophthalmic consultant performed a dilated fundus examination which revealed bilateral retinopathy in addition to disc edema. Retinal hemorrhages, cotton-wool spots and hard exudates were seen throughout the posterior poles, and macular edema was present in both eyes (Figure 1.4). A diagnosis of malignant hypertension was made and the patient was hospitalized for evaluation and initiation of treatment. Upon discharge, blood pressure control was maintained with oral medication and, at follow-up one month later, he reported resolution of headache and improvement of visual blur. Visual acuity was 20/25 in both eyes (OU) and there was marked improvement of disc edema and retinopathy.

Discussion: This patient with malignant hypertension presented with recent onset of headache and bilateral disc edema, suggesting the presence of increased intracranial pressure (ICP). Characteristics of the headache associated with increased ICP are non-specific and are so similar to those of increased systemic blood pressure that the distinction cannot be made based on the history. Associated symptoms such as pulsatile tinnitus or transient visual obscurations may be present in both conditions. Furthermore, both disorders can produce bilateral optic disc edema. The most important clue to the mechanism of disc edema in this case was the pattern of accompanying retinal abnormalities. Fully developed papilledema due to increased ICP may be accompanied by nerve fiber layer hemorrhages and exudates, but these vascular abnormalities are confined to the optic disc surface or the immediate peri-papillary nerve fiber layer (Figure 1.5A). The one exception is the occasional case in which hard exudates track from the swollen disc to form a partial macular star. As a general rule, the presence of retinal hemorrhages or exudates *beyond* one disc diameter from the optic nerve head indicates that a mechanism other than increased ICP underlies the disc edema (Figure 1.5B). The two main considerations in this setting are malignant hypertension and diabetes. The key feature that would have distinguished vascular disease of the eye from neurologic disease in this case was missed because a dilated fundus examination was not performed. Pharmacologic dilation is not contraindicated in a patient with disc edema who has no focal neurologic deficits and intact mental status.

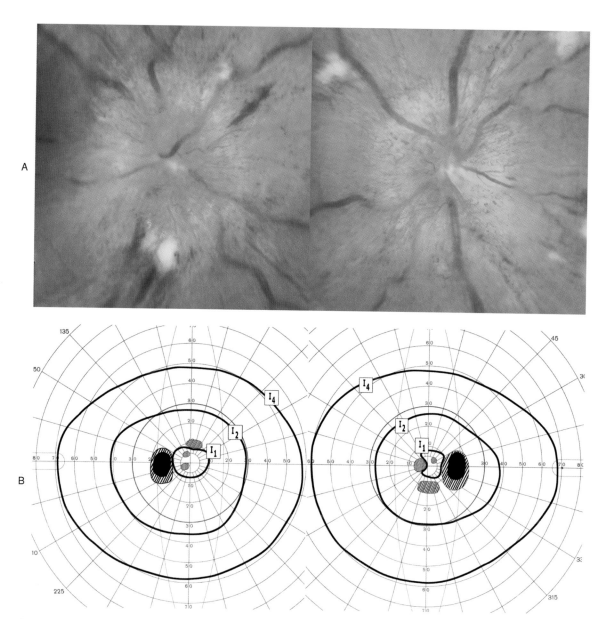

Figure 1.3 Examination findings in a 37-year-old schoolbus driver with daily headaches. (A) Both discs are diffusely swollen and hyperemic. Several nerve fiber layer (splinter) hemorrhages and cotton-wool spots are also present. (B) Goldmann perimetry shows bilateral central depression and small paracentral scotomas. The physiologic blindspot is also enlarged in each eye.

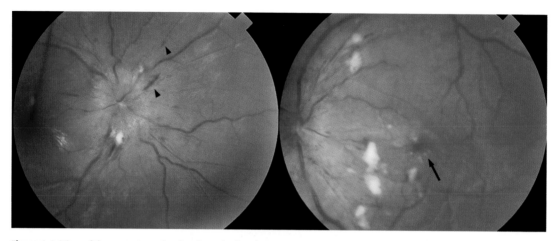

Figure 1.4 View of the posterior pole of each eye in the above patient. In addition to the previously noted optic disc edema, it is now apparent that the vascular abnormalities are not confined to the optic discs. Nerve fiber layer hemorrhages extend along the vascular arcades (arrowheads, right eye) and there are scattered cotton-wool spots throughout the posterior pole in the left eye. Macular edema is present in both eyes and small clumps of hard exudates can be seen in the parafoveal area (arrow). The arterioles are irregular and narrowed and the veins appear mildly engorged in both eyes.

A pronounced and sudden rise in blood pressure beyond the compensatory capacity of vascular autoregulation can result in vascular leakiness and widespread end-organ dysfunction affecting the brain, heart and kidney, a condition termed *malignant hypertension*. If untreated, such systemic involvement can cause irreversible tissue damage including myocardial infarction and stroke, and thus represents a true medical emergency. Retinal changes are the earliest ophthalmic abnormality associated with accelerated hypertension (Figure 1.6). Hemorrhages can be intraretinal (described as "dot/blot") or in the nerve fiber layer (termed "flame" or "splinter" hemorrhages) and are especially prominent along the vascular arcades. Occlusion of choroidal vessels may cause areas of secondary retinal detachment that can be focal or widespread. Later these areas may appear as retinal pigment atrophy or clumping, termed Elschnig spots. Macular alterations include edema, formation of microcysts and exudates. Nerve fiber layer infarcts appear as "cotton-wool spots" on the optic disc or the retina. Exudation in the retina may appear as punctate white opacities (indicating

focal pericapillary leakage) and hard exudates which may form a macular star figure. Malignant hypertension with disc edema and macular star formation is sometimes mistakenly diagnosed as bilateral neuroretinitis. Neuroretinitis rarely affects both eyes simultaneously and does not cause the more widespread retinal abnormalities found in malignant hypertension. In any patient thought to have bilateral acute neuroretinitis, it is mandatory to check the blood pressure. The pathogenesis of optic disc swelling in malignant hypertension is multifactorial, sometimes occurring as part of the retinopathy (due to vascular leakiness), in some cases representing ischemia of the optic nerve head and in others reflecting increased ICP (see below). Thus, disc edema may occur in the absence of observable retinopathy, and in such cases may be easily confused with papilledema of increased ICP.

Patients with malignant hypertension sometimes develop symptoms of cerebral dysfunction such as lethargy, confusion, seizures and focal neurologic deficits due to vascular changes in the brain, termed *hypertensive encephalopathy*. Extravasation of fluid

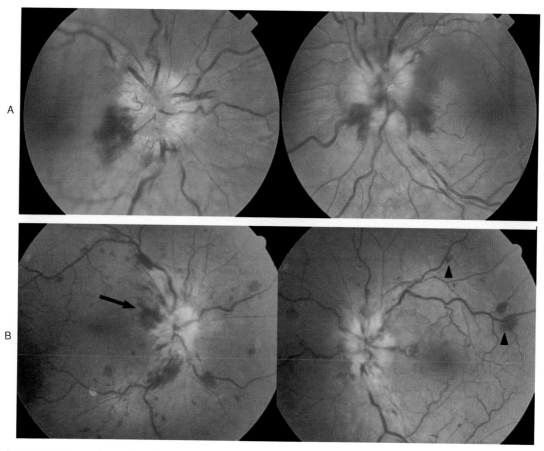

Figure 1.5 Patterns of hemorrhage in increased intracranial pressure vs. increased systemic blood pressure. (A) In papilledema (increased intracranial pressure) nerve fiber layer hemorrhages are limited to the disc and immediate peri-papillary region. (B) In malignant systemic hypertension the disc edema and peri-papillary hemorrhages (arrow) are similar, but these superficial hemorrhages also extend into the mid-peripheral retina. In addition there are intraretinal dot and blot hemorrhages throughout the posterior pole (arrowheads).

and protein from the intravascular space into the interstitium leads to vasogenic brain edema, which causes both cerebral dysfunction and increased intracranial pressure. In such patients, both ocular and neurologic pathology may contribute to disc swelling. Visual loss may similarly be due to both retinal and occipital cortical changes. The cerebral edema in this condition has a predilection for the parietal and occipital lobes and has been termed "posterior reversible encephalopathy syndrome". This condition is best demonstrated

on MR FLAIR sequences. In more severe cases, ischemic changes may also be seen on diffusion weighted images, which may progress to infarction and thus carry a more guarded prognosis. In pregnant women with acute hypertension, the same combination of clinical and radiographic findings is called the preeclampsia–eclampsia syndrome.

The clinical features and fundus findings in malignant hypertension are non-specific and may resemble several other conditions. Careful measurement of blood pressure should therefore be

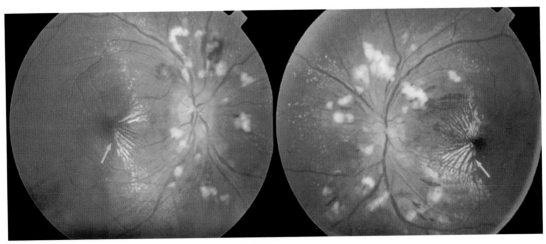

Figure 1.6 Fundus photographs of a different patient with retinovascular changes of malignant hypertension. Cotton-wool spots are present on the disc and along the vascular arcades. Scattered retinal flame and blot hemorrhages are seen in the same distribution. Hard exudates are found temporal to the optic disc, forming a partial macular star (arrows).

included in the evaluation of any patient with unexplained bilateral optic disc edema. With timely diagnosis and treatment, the clinical manifestations of malignant hypertension are often reversible. Overly rapid lowering of blood pressure, however, may cause devastating infarction of the optic nerves and other end organs and should be discouraged.

Diagnosis: Malignant hypertension

Tip: The presence of vascular changes in the retina distinguishes the optic disc swelling of malignant hypertension from that of increased intracranial pressure.

Chronic optic neuropathy

Case: A 40-year-old farmer noted blurring of vision in his left eye, of uncertain duration. He was generally healthy with no history of systemic or neurologic disease. There was a remote history of visual loss in the left eye due to trauma and he knew that vision in that eye hadn't returned to normal, but he wasn't certain if it had declined further since. Visual

acuity and color vision were normal in each eye. Visual field testing was normal in the right eye but markedly abnormal in the left (Figure 1.7). Ophthalmoscopic examination showed left optic disc pallor, which prompted an MR scan of brain and orbits that was normal.

Having excluded compressive, inflammatory and infiltrative causes of optic neuropathy, what other mechanisms would you consider? How would you proceed?

The pattern of this patient's visual field loss indicates damage at the level of the optic disc. Specifically, the defects emerge from the physiologic blindspot and respect the horizontal meridian. Common disc-related disorders include ischemic optic neuropathy, papilledema, disc drusen and glaucoma. The next step is a critical scrutiny of the optic disc.

The right disc has a normal appearance with a 0.2 cup/disc (C/D) ratio and healthy neuroretinal rim. The left disc, however, is severely excavated with virtually no neuroretinal rim (Figure 1.8).

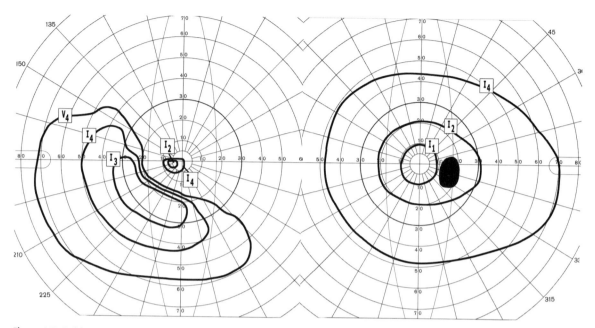

Figure 1.7 Goldmann visual field in a 40-year-old farmer. In the left eye there is a dense superior altitudinal defect coalescing with an inferior arcuate scotoma; the field in the right eye is normal.

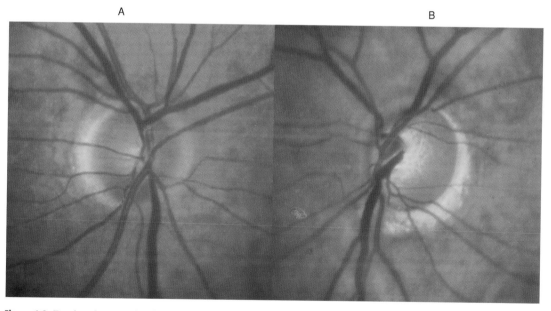

Figure 1.8 Fundus photographs of the above patient with severe visual field loss in the left eye. (A) The right optic disc is normal. (B) The left optic disc is markedly cupped, leaving almost no neuroretinal rim. Even without a stereoscopic view, the deep saucerization can be appreciated from the curve of the retinal vessels as they emerge from the cup and cross the disc margin. The stippled appearance in the center of the disc indicates that this is the lamina cribrosa, and not neural tissue.

Its pale color is misleading. What the viewer is seeing is exposed lamina cribrosa, which, being a continuation of the sclera, is normally white. Based on this optic disc appearance, ophthalmic consultation was obtained. His intraocular pressures (IOPs) were asymmetric, measuring 13 mm OD and 26 mm OS. Gonioscopy revealed angle recession in the left eye, presumed due to his past history of eye injury. He was treated with topical medications to lower the IOP in his left eye, and subsequent serial examinations showed that his visual field defect was stable.

Discussion: The optic disc has a limited repertoire of expression. Processes that interfere with axonal transport cause disc swelling, whereas those that reflect axonal loss manifest as pallor and/or excavation. Acquired excavation of the optic nerve head, or disc cupping, is traditionally divided into glaucomatous and non-glaucomatous forms. The large majority of cases of disc cupping are glaucomatous in origin.

Glaucomatous optic nerve damage has a characteristic appearance. The disease has a predilection for the arcuate fibers, which produces progressive loss of the neural rim starting at the superior and inferior poles of the optic disc, and causes vertical elongation of the cup. If both eyes are equally affected, this early stage of the disease may be difficult to recognize. In other cases, asymmetry of the C/D ratio in the two eyes may be the first sign of the condition (Figure 1.9A). An interocular C/D asymmetry of 0.1 or more is found in only 10% of the normal population, and thus raises suspicion of glaucoma. Another helpful finding is the presence of a single splinter hemorrhage on the disc margin, termed a Drance hemorrhage (Figure 1.9B). While similar hemorrhages are seen in a variety of conditions that cause disc edema, in the absence of disc swelling this finding is strongly suggestive of glaucoma. Focal damage to the nerve fiber layer, appearing as a notch in the neural rim, is also characteristic of glaucomatous optic neuropathy and sometimes follows a Drance hemorrhage (Figure 1.9C).

Uncommonly, causes of optic nerve damage other than glaucoma produce optic disc excavation.

These mechanisms include compression, disc infarction due to giant cell arteritis, trauma and radiation necrosis. The fundus feature that is most helpful for distinguishing glaucomatous from non-glaucomatous cupping is the status of the remaining neural rim. In glaucomatous discs, the rim generally maintains a more normal hue. Even in advanced cases of glaucoma in which nerve fiber loss is severe, the degree of disc excavation is disproportionately greater than the severity of rim pallor (Figure 1.10). In contrast, rim pallor is a prominent feature of non-glaucomatous cupping. Other fundus features may also be helpful in making this distinction. Focal thinning of the temporal retinal rim is more characteristic of non-glaucomatous damage, whereas diffuse obliteration of the neural rim and peri-papillary atrophy usually reflect glaucomatous change.

In addition to optic disc appearance, measures of optic nerve function are also important. In keeping with the predilection for superior and inferior nerve fiber bundles, field defects in glaucoma are typically arcuate, particularly affecting the superior field. Central vision is spared until late in the course of the disease. In contrast, compressive causes of acquired disc excavation are often associated with visual field loss that respects the vertical meridian. The clinical challenge in cases such as the above is to distinguish optic disc excavation from disc atrophy. Despite advances in optic disc imaging techniques such as ocular coherence tomography (OCT), careful fundus examination is usually the key to making this diagnosis.

Diagnosis: Glaucomatous optic neuropathy

Tip: Glaucoma should be included in the differential diagnosis for any patient with unexplained optic neuropathy.

Painful mydriasis

Case: A 62-year-old librarian periodically noted a dull pain around her right eye when she worked nights in the archives section. At times, along with

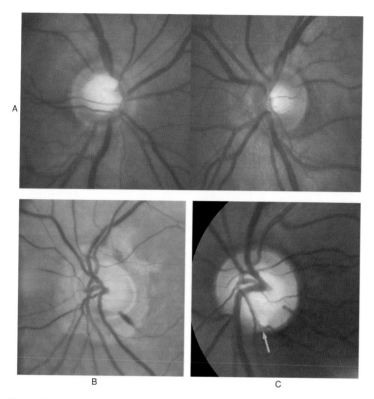

Figure 1.9 Examples of glaucomatous optic disc changes. (A) Greater loss of nerve fiber layer in the right eye results in asymmetric cupping. The C/D ratio in the right eye is 0.7 compared to a 0.4 C/D ratio in the left eye. (B) Peri-papillary pigment disturbance and a characteristic Drance (splinter) hemorrhage at the inferotemporal disc margin. (C) Focal excavation of the neural rim inferiorly (arrow).

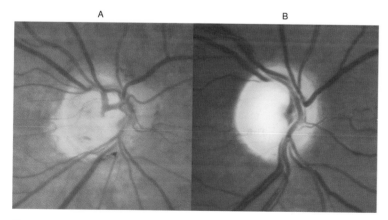

Figure 1.10 Comparison of glaucomatous vs. non-glaucomatous disc excavation. (A) Despite severe cupping due to glaucoma, the remaining neural rim retains a nearly normal color. (B) Following optic nerve trauma, this disc shows cupping and severe pallor of the remaining neural rim.

the pain she experienced fuzziness of vision and halos around lights in her right eye. Her symptoms always resolved by the following morning so she did not seek medical advice until one evening when her dull pain rapidly escalated to a severe right-sided headache. She felt weak and nauseated and could not see well. In the emergency room, visual acuity was 20/60 OD and 20/20 OS. There was mild aniso-coria in room light (right pupil 4.5 mm compared to left pupil 3.5 mm), and the right pupil was non-reactive to light and near stimulation. Eye move-ments were full and there was no ptosis. Before any further examination could be performed, she became bradycardic and hypotensive and vomited. Acute third nerve palsy due to ruptured posterior communicating artery (pCOM) aneurysm was sus-pected, and she was sent for immediate brain MRI and magnetic resonance angiography (MRA). These imaging studies, however, were normal.

What clues suggest an alternative diagnosis?

The first clue is the unilateral pupillary unreactiv-ity in the absence of other neurologic deficits. When the pupil is dysfunctional due to a pCOM aneurysm, it is virtually always associated with other elements of a third nerve palsy (NP). In the setting of transten-torial herniation, a dilated pupil is occasionally the earliest sign of third nerve compression, but in such cases there is also alteration of consciousness and, in most cases, other focal neurologic deficits. The presence of an *isolated*, non-reactive pupil in an awake patient should be considered an indication of ocular rather than intracranial disease. The sec-ond and more specific clue that helps to further narrow the differential is the patient's description of seeing halos in the eye with the mydriasis. This symptom is not due to the pupillary unresponsive-ness but indicates, in addition, an aberration of the ocular media. In this patient, the most likely cause is corneal edema secondary to *acute angle closure glaucoma*.

After her negative neuro-imaging, an ophthalmic consultant confirmed an elevated intraocular pres-sure of 55 mmHg in the right eye and closure of the

angle. Examination also revealed mild conjunctival injection and corneal haze (Figure 1.11). The patient was treated with acetazolamide, timolol and pilo-carpine followed by anterior chamber paracentesis, which brought dramatic relief of pain. She subse-quently underwent bilateral peripheral laser irido-tomies and has had no further attacks of pain.

Discussion: Angle closure glaucoma can be cate-gorized as primary (due to a structurally narrow angle) or secondary (due to inflammation, trauma, ischemia or other ocular disorders). In secondary glaucoma the examination typically shows evidence of the condition that produced the changes in the drainage system. In contrast, in patients with primary angle closure the examination between episodes may be entirely normal and thus the diag-nosis may be more challenging.

The clinical manifestations of angle closure glau-coma are variable with some patients hardly symp-tomatic and others nearly prostrate with pain. Many patients have repeated self-limited episodes of sub-acute angle closure before a full attack. Such pro-dromal attacks generally consist of unilateral face or head pain accompanied by blurred vision and halos around lights, typically lasting 30–60 minutes. Pain is usually localized around the eye but may extend to the maxillary region and mimic dental pathol-ogy. In occasional patients, headache rather than eye pain is the presenting symptom. Because there is often conjunctival injection during an attack, these painful episodes may be mistaken for clus-ter headache or other hemi-cranial headache syn-dromes. It is important that neurologists keep the possibility of angle closure attacks in the differ-ential diagnosis for these patients and consider ophthalmic referral to evaluate this possibility in selected patients.

Factors that may precipitate an attack in predis-posed individuals include prone position, a dark or dim light environment, prolonged near-work, stress, sneezing, pharmacologic mydriasis and cer-tain anesthetic agents. Patients with a high degree of hyperopia are particularly prone to such attacks. During an attack of angle closure, the IOP increases

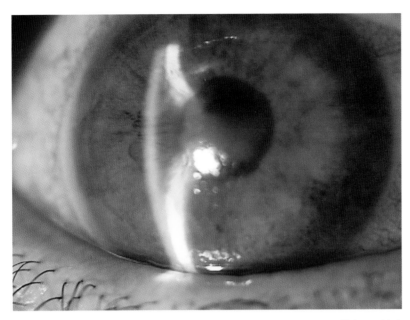

Figure 1.11 A 62-year-old woman with recurrent unilateral headache, visual blur and halos around lights. Slit-lamp photograph shows mild conjunctival hyperemia, corneal haze and forward bowing of the iris consistent with acute angle closure glaucoma. (Photograph courtesy of Dr. Emilie Ravinet.)

rapidly and is accompanied by conjunctival injection and corneal edema due to hypoxia and secondary corneal decompensation. The pupil is midsize and fixed. In subacute cases, the angle reopens spontaneously and symptoms and signs resolve. Between attacks the examination is usually normal although careful inspection will often reveal the narrow angle that predisposes to acute closure. The diagnosis is established by gonioscopy or ultrasound biomicroscopy. Although assessment of intraocular pressure by digital examination is generally considered to be unreliable, this technique may be useful in cases with markedly elevated pressures when biomicroscopy is not immediately available.

When the onset of pain is explosive and accompanied by a vasovagal reaction and vomiting, as was the case above, the clinical scenario mimics acute intracranial pathology. The presence of a dilated pupil further adds to the impression of a cerebral aneurysm. It is important that neurologists keep

the possibility of acute angle closure glaucoma in the differential diagnosis of painful isolated mydriasis and seek urgent ophthalmic referral in selected patients before proceeding with neurologic investigations.

Diagnosis: Acute angle closure glaucoma

Tip: Acute angle closure glaucoma causes acute headache and an unreactive pupil. A history of blurred vision with halos in the eye with mydriasis suggests the diagnosis.

Invisible retinal disease

In most cases, retinal disease can be detected by a thorough dilated fundus examination. Occasionally, however, such abnormalities are absent either due to the nature of the disease process, the timing of the examination or the expertise of the examiner. In these cases the absence of apparent retinal abnormality may create the impression of neurologic disease. The cases that follow are examples of such occult retinal disorders.

In some cases of "invisible" retinal disease, the diagnosis becomes apparent with fluorescein angiography. An example of this is Stargardt's disease. Many macular disorders that at one time would have been considered occult are now readily identified with optical coherence tomography (OCT). Common examples in this category include central serous choroidopathy and cystoid macular edema. In some conditions in which the fundus examination and fluorescein angiographic findings may be normal, the pathology can be demonstrated with electrophysiology. The full-field electroretinogram (ERG) is abnormal in paraneoplastic retinopathies, retinitis pigmentosa and in vitamin A deficiency; however certain other disorders can be demonstrated only with multi-focal ERG. Examples of the latter include outer retinal inflammatory diseases and some toxic maculopathies such as that induced by chloroquine.

The importance of recognizing the symptoms and other clinical features that indicate a retinal disorder is in knowing when to employ these ancillary tests.

Twinkling scotoma

Case: A 25-year-old female graduate student sought medical attention because of a one-month history of scintillations. Specifically, she described a dark, oval-shaped spot temporal to fixation in her right eye, with continuous sparkling at its edge. She compared the appearance of this sparkling to that of "the sun reflecting off the rippled surface of a lake". She had noticed no change in the size or shape of the spot since onset and there was no associated head or eye pain. She was generally healthy and her only medication was oral contraceptives. General eye examination was unrevealing and an MRI of the brain was also normal. She was started on topiramate for presumed migraine, but her twinkling scotoma persisted.

What aspect of this patient's positive visual phenomenon is highly atypical for migraine?

While migraine is a common cause of photopsias, the *continuous* nature of this patient's scintillations would be highly unusual. Another atypical aspect of the history is the monocular nature of her scotoma. However, it should be noted that many patients with episodic visual disturbance involving one hemifield interpret their visual deficit as affecting just the eye with the temporal field defect. In such cases it is helpful to ask the patient what they can and cannot see during the attack. Inability to see one half of an object (such as a face or a clock) is inconsistent with monocular loss and indicates instead a homonymous hemifield deficit. In the above case, the examiner verified that the visual disturbance was truly monocular.

Subsequent neuro-ophthalmic examination demonstrated normal visual acuity, pupillary responses and fundus appearance. Goldmann perimetry showed marked enlargement of the physiologic blindspot in the right eye. A multi-focal electroretinogram (mfERG) revealed decreased amplitude in the corresponding area of the right eye (Figure 1.12). Based on these findings, a diagnosis of *acute idiopathic blindspot enlargement* (AIBSE) was made.

The patient was followed expectantly and over the next several years the blindspot in her right eye became smaller but the sparkling continued. Ten years later, she still noted persistent scintillations in the involved area but found that they did not interfere with her daily activities. The peri-papillary retina in that eye had now developed a mottled, grayish appearance (Figure 1.13).

Discussion: Photopsias are a form of positive visual phenomenon that can arise anywhere along the afferent visual pathway. Several clinical features are helpful in localizing their origin. Photopsias that are evoked by eye movement indicate a disorder in the anterior part of the visual system, usually due to vitreous traction, retinal detachment or optic neuritis. The last of these is typically associated with

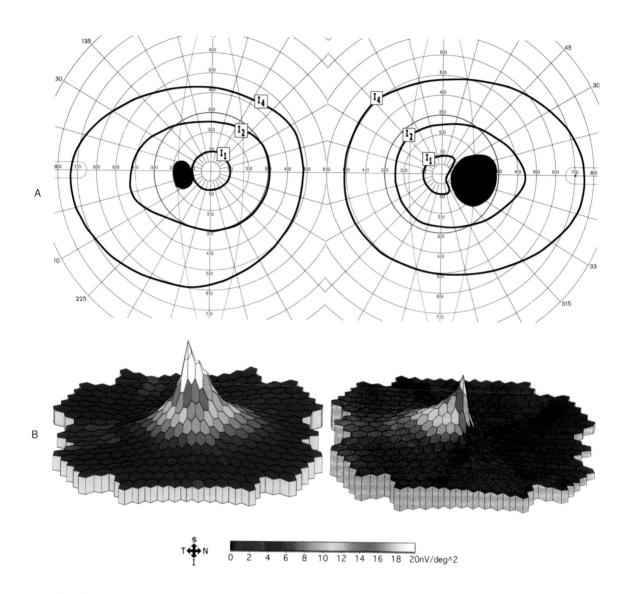

Figure 1.12 Visual testing in the above young woman with a persistent twinkling scotoma. (A) Goldmann perimetry shows enlargement of the physiologic blindspot in the right eye to nearly four times the normal-sized blindspot in the left eye. (B) The three-dimensional plot of a multi-focal ERG (mfERG) is normal in the left eye and shows marked reduction of the response density surrounding the physiologic blindspot in the right eye, corresponding to the patient's scotoma.

pain, whereas vitreous and retinal detachments are not. In cases of spontaneous photopsias, the pattern of visual loss can suggest the correct localization, hence the utility of formal visual field testing in patients with this symptom. Occipital disorders are a frequent source of positive visual phenomena, including photopsias. The three main diagnostic considerations in this location are migraine, transient ischemic attacks (TIAs) and occipital seizures.

A   B

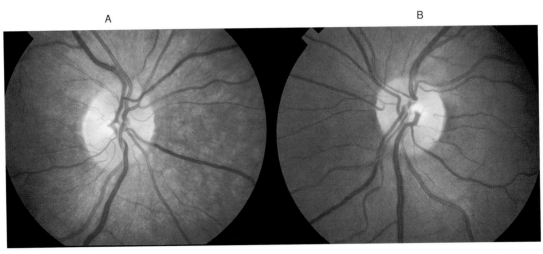

Figure 1.13 Fundus photographs of the same patient 10 years later. The previously enlarged blindspot had gradually diminished but she continued to experience photopsias in the right eye. (A) The peri-papillary retina in the right eye now has a grayish, moth-eaten appearance. (B) The left fundus is normal.

Migraine visual aura usually consists of scintillations that are geometric and achromatic lasting 20 to 30 minutes (see Chapter 11, Episodic scintillating scotoma). Transient ischemia affecting the vertebrobasilar circulation tends to produce negative visual symptoms, but occasional attacks include a positive visual element, sometimes compared to "the appearance of snow falling through the beam of a headlight". Such TIAs last a few minutes and may be accompanied by other focal neurologic deficits. Occipital seizures may resemble migraine aura but are generally shorter in duration, lasting for 5 minutes or less, and often consist of colored circles rather than the achromatic zigzags of migraine. Occipital seizures may be accompanied by alteration of awareness and by automatisms such as frequent blinking or gaze deviation. Regardless of the mechanism, the duration of positive visual phenomena emanating from the occipital cortex is finite. With rare exceptions, after about 30 minutes the occipital lobe "wears out" and photopsias cease.

This is not the case for the outer retina. Any metabolic failure involving photoreceptors or retinal pigment epithelium cells can result in positive phenomena such as flashing lights, shimmers and sparkles, which can persist indefinitely. This is because photoreceptors are normally in a depolarized state, becoming hyperpolarized in response to a light stimulus. Energy failure of any cause can result in an inability to maintain depolarization and thus the production of light flashes. Specific etiologies include retinitis pigmentosa, paraneoplastic retinopathies, toxic retinopathies and a spectrum of presumed inflammatory disorders of the outer retina. The latter disorders are sometimes classified under the term *acute zonal occult outer retinopathy* (AZOOR).

The common feature in all of the AZOOR syndromes is a dense, sharply demarcated scotoma which appears acutely in any portion of the visual field with minimal or no fundus abnormalities. Photopsias, which may antedate or follow the visual loss, are present in almost 90% of cases. Individual descriptions of the photopsia include terms like light flashes, stars, strobe lights, sparkling, whirling, shimmering or flickering. In acute idiopathic blindspot enlargement the fundamental feature is a dense, steeply margined scotoma centered around the physiologic blindspot, as in the above

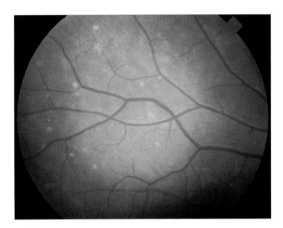

Figure 1.14 Fundus photograph of a patient with MEWDS, showing the characteristic lesions in the mid-peripheral retina.

case. The peri-papillary retina is the target of inflammation, and the focal area of disturbed photoreceptor function is best demonstrated with multi-focal rather than full-field ERG. In the acute stage, the fundus is normal save for mild optic nerve swelling in some patients. Multiple evanescent white dot syndrome (MEWDS), a closely related syndrome, is characterized in its acute stage by small whitish lesions in the posterior pole (Figure 1.14), and may also be associated with a persistently enlarged blindspot.

The etiology of AIBSE is unknown. The disorder usually affects healthy young women, and evaluation discloses no evidence of an underlying systemic disease. There is no established treatment but the natural history usually includes spontaneous improvement of the scotoma, although photopsias may persist.

As in the above case, prominent photopsias in patients with AIBSE may be mistaken for the visual disturbance of migraine. Because this disorder presents as acute onset of a monocular scotoma, it may also suggest a diagnosis of demyelinating optic neuritis. The absence of pain and the continuous nature of the scintillations are important distinguishing features.

Diagnosis: Acute idiopathic blindspot enlargement

Tip: Continuous photopsias indicate a disorder of the outer retina.

Sudden monocular visual loss with normal fundus

Case: This 70-year-old gentleman experienced sudden, painless visual loss in the left eye while watching television. At the onset of his visual loss he saw an arc of yellow lights briefly passing across the superior visual field in the left eye. He was generally healthy except for prostate cancer for which he was taking diethylstilbesterol. Examination in a local emergency room within six hours after onset of visual loss showed 20/20 acuity in the right eye (OD) and count fingers vision in the left eye (OS), but revealed no basis for his acute visual loss. Based on the normal fundus appearance, he was thought to have a retrobulbar optic neuropathy, but an MRI of brain and orbits was completely normal.

What other mechanism of visual loss would you consider? Are there any historical features that are helpful here?

A compressive or infiltrative optic nerve lesion should be in the differential, however the very abrupt onset of visual loss in this case would be unusual and his MRI was unrevealing. Optic neuritis is a possibility, but the patient's age would be highly atypical for demyelinating disease. Acute painless monocular visual loss in a patient over the age of 50 years is most often ischemic in origin, and that should be the main consideration in this case. The question is whether this ischemia affects the optic nerve or the retina. In the large majority of cases, ischemic optic neuropathy affects the most anterior portion of the nerve so that disc edema is seen acutely, termed *anterior ischemic optic neuropathy* (AION). In this patient, however, the disc was normal. Ischemia of the retrobulbar segment of the optic nerve, termed *posterior ischemic optic neuropathy* (PION), is rare. When PION does occur, it is generally in the setting of severe prolonged hypotension, often accompanied by blood loss (e.g. peri-operative, cardiac arrest or massive hemorrhage) or due to giant cell arteritis. A diagnosis of PION in any other setting should be suspect. In addition, the presence of photopsias heralding the onset of visual loss would be highly unusual in either form of ischemic optic neuropathy but sometimes accompanies a retinal ischemic event. Retinal artery occlusion is therefore the leading diagnosis in this case.

Why might a retinal stroke not have been apparent on examination?

Retinal whitening due to arterial occlusion may take up to 24 hours to develop. Other fundus features related to lack of flow in the retinal circulation, such as ghost vessels and segmentation of the blood column (termed "boxcarring") in retinal arteries may be seen hyperacutely, but if flow has been restored in the occluded vessel the fundus may have a completely normal appearance during this interval.

Based on the above considerations, the patient was treated presumptively for *central retinal artery occlusion* (CRAO) including ocular massage, anterior chamber paracentesis, oxygen/carbon dioxide breathing and acetazolamide. Ophthalmic examination three days later showed no change of visual acuity in the left eye. There was a large central scotoma and small relative afferent pupillary defect (RAPD). Dilated fundus examination now showed retinal whitening (edema) of the posterior pole with a macular cherry-red spot, confirming a diagnosis of CRAO (Figure 1.15). Ancillary investigation revealed no embolic source, and testing for vasculitis and coagulation disorders was similarly unrevealing. His CRAO was attributed to a hypercoaguable state secondary to treatment with diethystilbesterol.

Discussion: Retinal artery occlusion typically produces acute, painless, monocular visual loss. Unlike individuals with ischemic optic neuropathy, who often note visual loss upon awakening, patients

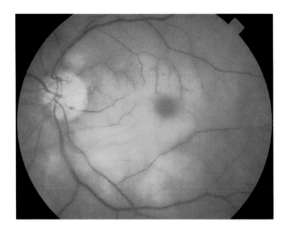

Figure 1.15 Fundus photograph of the above 70-year-old man with acute painless visual loss in his left eye three days previously. There is diffuse retinal whitening and a cherry-red spot in the macula, indicating central retinal artery occlusion.

with retinal artery occlusion can often describe just what they were doing when visual loss occurred. Permanent visual loss due to retinal artery occlusion is sometimes preceded by episodes of transient monocular visual loss, usually lasting for less than five minutes, often with an altitudinal pattern described as a "curtain" descending over vision. In contrast, such episodes of preceding transient monocular visual loss are distinctly uncommon in patients with non-arteritic AION.

The fundus appearance in retinal artery occlusion depends on the timing of the examination. In the hyperacute phase there may be obvious attenuation and segmentation of the blood column within retinal arteries, and the responsible embolus may be visible. If the embolic material has moved on through the retinal circulation, however, and flow has already been restored, the retina may have a completely normal appearance. This phase may last up to 24 hours. As edema develops, areas of retinal whitening appear. This may take the form of cotton-wool spots (indicating small nerve fiber infarcts) or of patchy or diffuse retinal whitening. The distribution of retinal edema varies depending on whether the central or a branch retinal artery was involved (Figure 1.16). In cases of central retinal artery

A   B

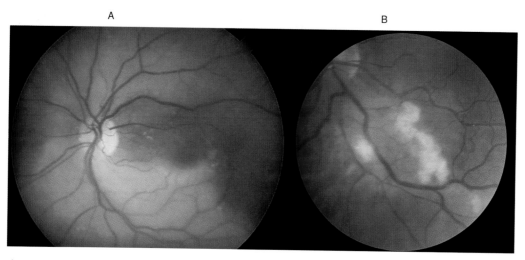

Figure 1.16 Retinal changes associated with branch retinal artery occlusion. (A) There is a sharp demarcation between the area of acute retinal infarction, which appears white due to edema, and the normal adjacent retina. (B) Confluent cotton-wool spots represent focal infarcts of the nerve fiber layer.

occlusion, the entire posterior retina is thickened and white except for a central cherry-red spot which is due to preserved flow in the choroidal circulation that supplies this area. In the chronic phase, after retinal edema has resolved, differentiating between retinal and optic nerve ischemia may again be difficult. Because of retrograde axonal degeneration, in the wake of a retinovascular event the optic disc will appear pale, either focally or diffusely. In this stage, electrophysiologic testing, usually with the mfERG, can be helpful for making this distinction.

Diagnosis: Hyperacute central retinal artery occlusion

Tip: In a hyperacute retinal artery occlusion, the retina may have a normal appearance.

Hazy night vision

Case: Over a six-month period this 55-year-old postal worker noticed slowly progressive "haziness" of vision in both eyes, especially in dim illumination. This became so severe that he started using a nightlight and stopped driving after dark. He had no head or eye pain, focal neurologic deficits or systemic symptoms. His medical history

was positive for hypertension, hypercholesterolemia and previous morbid obesity for which he had undergone gastric bypass surgery 12 years earlier. Visual acuity was 20/25 OU with normal color vision and pupillary responses. Goldmann perimetry showed mild superior depression, and dilated fundus examination was normal (Figure 1.17). A fluorescein angiogram and ocular coherence tomography (OCT) were also unrevealing. Based on the negative ophthalmic work-up, a neurologic cause was suspected and the patient was referred for neurologic evaluation. An MRI showed a few white matter lesions consistent with small vessel disease but was otherwise normal.

What specific aspect of this patient's history suggests the correct localization of his visual problem?

Difficulty seeing at night (nyctalopia) strongly suggests retinal disease, specifically a disorder of photoreceptors preferentially involving the rods. In this patient, a full-field electroretinogram (ERG) showed markedly reduced amplitudes on scotopic testing and mild reduction on photopic testing, confirming rod dysfunction (Figure 1.18A). A serum retinol

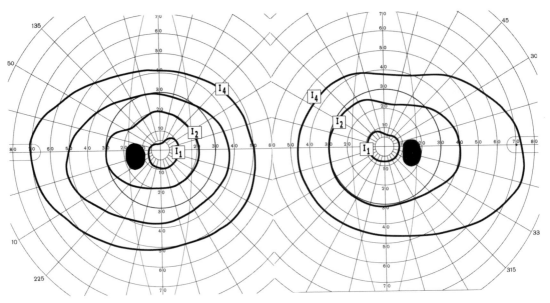

Figure 1.17 Goldmann perimetry in a 55-year-old postal worker with decreased night vision. There is mild superior depression affecting central and mid-peripheral isopters in both eyes.

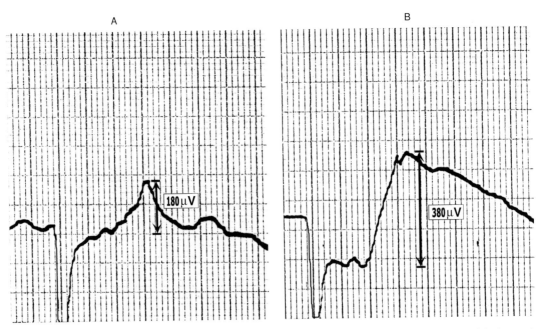

Figure 1.18 Full-field scotopic ERG in the left eye of the above patient. (A) At initial testing, the amplitude of the b-wave is decreased at 180 μV. (B) Following treatment with vitamin A the b-wave amplitude has increased to 380 μV.

(vitamin A) level was reduced at 0.09 mg/L (normal 0.30–1.20). The patient received a diagnosis of retinal dysfunction due to hypovitaminosis A related to prior gastric bypass surgery. He was treated with 100 000 units of oral vitamin A per day, and over the next six weeks experienced progressive recovery of vision. A repeat ERG showed an increase in the scotopic amplitudes bilaterally (Figure 1.18B).

Discussion: Vitamin A is a fat-soluble vitamin that is absorbed across the small intestinal mucosa and transported to the liver, where it is stored in its esterified form (retinol) and available in protein-bound form to reach target tissues. In the retina it is stored in the retinal pigment epithelial cells and converted to the aldehyde form (retinal), which then combines with opsin to form rhodopsin. Vitamin A deficiency can result from inadequate nutritional intake (common in underdeveloped countries), poor intestinal absorption, impaired liver storage capacity or inadequate enzymatic conversion of retinol to retinal (a process that is dependent upon zinc as a co-factor). Causes of malabsorption include intestinal bypass surgery, regional enteritis and cystic fibrosis. Liver disease may cause hypovitaminosis A by a variety of mechanisms: decreased production of retinol-binding protein, inadequate storage of retinol, malabsorption due to decreased bile salts and depletion of zinc stores. Occasionally, deficiency is caused by the use of a synthetic vitamin A analog such as isotretinoin.

Ophthalmic manifestations of vitamin A deficiency typically include dry eyes and retinopathy. The earliest symptom is usually nyctalopia due to the greater dependency of rods on rapid transport with retinal pigment epithelial (RPE) cells. If the deficiency is not corrected, this is followed by visual field loss, photophobia and decreased acuity. Severe loss of visual acuity and color vision is unusual. Visual field testing may show central and paracentral defects that affect the superior field more than the inferior field.

Funduscopic examination is often normal, especially in early vitamin A deficiency, thus causing confusion with neurologic visual loss. With pro-

longed deficiency, multiple yellowish-white dots may appear in the mid-peripheral retina, giving it a stippled appearance. Fluorescein angiography may demonstrate numerous punctate RPE defects which correspond to these retinal lesions. These clinical abnormalities are present to varying degrees and are generally reversible within several months after vitamin repletion. Electrophysiologic tests such as dark adaptometry and full-field ERG are quite sensitive in this condition, revealing abnormal rod function even in the absence of visual symptoms. Eventually there is elevation of the threshold and loss of waveform amplitude for both rods and cones, though rod function is more severely affected. The diagnosis should be suspected on clinical grounds and confirmed by testing the vitamin A level. Following treatment, the electrophysiologic abnormalities are faster to improve than the fundus abnormalities, and the final visual prognosis is generally good although in cases of prolonged depletion permanent damage may occur.

Diagnosis: Hypovitaminosis A

Tip: Even in the absence of ophthalmoscopic abnormalities, a history of acquired, progressive nyctalopia should suggest a retinal disorder.

Swirling vision

Case: A 60-year-old plumber developed visual loss in the right eye accompanied by intermittent "swirling clouds of smoke" and occasional dim flashes of light. He did not have eye pain but did have prominent photophobia and noted that his vision was much worse in bright light. Visual acuity was count fingers OD and 20/25 OS. The visual field in the right eye showed a ring scotoma and was normal in the left eye. Dilated fundus examination and fluorescein angiography were normal. A retrobulbar optic neuropathy was suspected but an MRI of brain and orbits with gadolinium was normal. He received a tentative diagnosis of posterior ischemic optic neuropathy. Two months later, similar though milder visual loss developed in the left eye

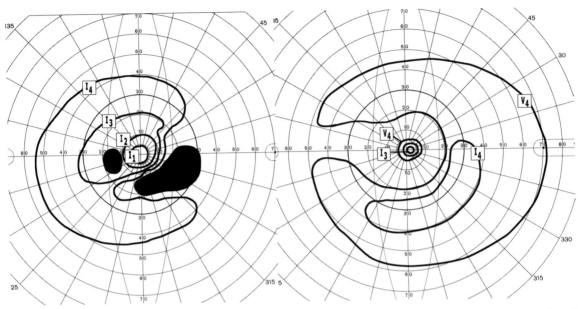

Figure 1.19 Goldmann perimetry in a 60-year-old plumber with bilateral sequential visual loss and photopsias. In the right eye there is a dense ring scotoma breaking out to the periphery. In the left eye there is an inferior arcuate scotoma that breaks out nasally.

(Figure 1.19). As before, the fundus appearance was normal.

A full-field ERG was nearly unrecordable under both scotopic and photopic conditions, indicating severe dysfunction of both rods and cones. Serologic testing showed antibodies to recoverin, diagnostic of cancer-associated retinopathy (CAR). A chest radiograph was normal but a chest computerized tomography (CT) scan revealed a small lesion which, on biopsy, proved to be a small cell lung carcinoma. His primary tumor was treated with radiation and chemotherapy and he received a course of high-dose intravenous corticosteroids followed by rituximab. Vision stabilized but unfortunately showed minimal improvement.

Discussion: *Cancer-associated retinopathy* (CAR) is a paraneoplastic syndrome in which antibodies directed toward a neoplasm also attack specific sites in the retina. It is most commonly associated with small cell lung carcinoma but has been described with various other malignancies including non-small cell lung cancer, breast and gynecologic malignancies, prostate and bladder cancer. In half of patients with the syndrome, the presence of a malignancy is unsuspected at the onset of visual loss. The typical presentation consists of subacute, bilateral visual deterioration associated with photopsias and a variety of other entoptic phenomena including swirls, clouds, smoke and floaters. Early in the disease, the fundus appearance is normal. Later, attenuated arterioles, mottling of the retinal pigment epithelium, disc pallor and vitreous cells may be seen. The triad of photosensitivity, ring scotomas and attenuated retinal arterioles, particularly in an older patient, should suggest a diagnosis of CAR syndrome.

The autoimmune mechanism of CAR has been established with the discovery of auto-antibodies directed toward retina-specific antigens. To date, more than 15 auto-antibodies to the retina have been identified. The most common is the anti-recoverin antibody, which targets a 23 kD protein (recoverin) found in rods and cones. As with other disorders of cones, visual function is worse in bright light (*hemeralopia*), and complaints of photophobia and glare are common. Visual field loss may initially reflect rod dysfunction (mid-peripheral defects and ring scotomas) but central loss soon ensues. The ERG is uniformly abnormal in CAR syndrome, usually showing loss of a- and b-waveforms under photopic and scotopic conditions. Even when central acuity is relatively preserved, the ERG may be surprisingly flat. While the electrophysiologic abnormalities in CAR are indistinguishable from those of some hereditary retinal dystrophies, the more rapid progression and older age at onset are features favoring a diagnosis of CAR syndrome.

As in the above case, the normal fundus appearance and fluorescein angiogram create the impression of neurologic visual loss. The abnormal ERG localizes the visual loss to the retina. The presence of auto-antibodies confirms the diagnosis, although such antibodies are not present in all cases. If the clinical findings suggest CAR, screening tests for occult malignancy should be undertaken, even in the absence of a positive antibody test. Treatment is aimed at eradicating or controlling the primary malignancy though corticosteroids, and other immunomodulatory therapies have also been used in an effort to prevent additional visual loss. In most cases reversal of visual loss is not possible.

Diagnosis: Cancer-associated retinopathy

Tip: Prominent degradation of vision in bright light (hemeralopia) suggests underlying retinal disease, particularly affecting cone function.

Episodic monocular blur

Case: This 65-year-old retired accountant described a one-month history of episodic visual loss in the right eye. Specifically, he noted blurring of vision lasting several hours, often present immediately upon awakening. After each episode his vision returned to baseline. There was no associated pain, photophobia or positive visual phenomena. He had undergone uncomplicated cataract extraction with intraocular lens implant in each eye one

year earlier. Ophthalmic and neurologic examination showed only mildly decreased visual acuity of 20/30 OU, attributed to capsular fibrosis and mild corneal guttatae. Subsequent evaluation included carotid Dopplers, MR angiography of the cervical vessels, erythrocyte sedimentation rate (ESR), C-reactive protein (CRP) and complete blood count (CBC), all of which were normal.

This patient's work-up addressed the possibility of retinal vascular disease as the cause of his transient monocular visual loss (TMVL). Is there something about his history, however, to suggest a different mechanism for his episodes?

This patient's history of visual loss that was present upon awakening even before arising from bed would be highly atypical for ischemia but quite characteristic of a particular corneal disorder. Corneal decompensation is often worse first thing in the morning because lid closure during the night prevents normal oxygenation and evaporation. This patient was asked to return for evaluation early in the day while experiencing the blurred vision. Examination of the right eye during an episode showed moderate edema of the corneal stroma with macrocystic epithelial changes. More detailed investigation showed his corneal thickness was increased at 670 μm and endothelial photography confirmed a reduced cell count of 500/mm. A diagnosis of *Fuchs corneal dystrophy* was made.

Discussion: A history of episodic visual loss prompts consideration of a neurovascular mechanism. The most common vascular cause of transient monocular visual loss (TMVL) is retinal embolism. Transient visual disturbance due to retinal emboli (also termed *amaurosis fugax*) typically has an abrupt onset and offset, often described as a curtain or shade descending over vision. Similar to hemispheric transient ischemic attacks, most episodes of TMVL due to embolic retinal ischemia last for just 5 to 10 minutes. Episodes are usually spontaneous and are not accompanied by pain. The source of retinal emboli is commonly the internal carotid artery, sometimes the heart and rarely the great vessels of the neck.

TMVL due to ischemia also occurs in the ocular ischemic syndrome (OIS). The mechanism of visual loss in this condition is different from that of retinal emboli, and thus the characteristics of the visual loss are different as well. Ocular ischemia most often occurs in the setting of high-grade carotid stenosis or occlusion and occasionally secondary to giant cell arteritis. Decreased perfusion can affect all ocular and orbital structures, causing ischemia of the anterior and posterior segments of the eye and extraocular muscles to varying degrees.

The visual loss in OIS is more gradual in onset and of longer duration compared to embolic visual episodes, often lasting minutes to hours. Visual loss in OIS is often precipitated by exposure to bright light or by postural change, with episodes induced by arising and relieved by lying down. Thus the history of transient visual loss in this condition might sound somewhat like that described by the above patient with corneal disease; however the important distinguishing feature is that in OIS visual loss begins only upon arising from bed, whereas in corneal decompensation vision is blurry as soon as the individual awakens. In contrast to patients with embolic TMVL, patients with OIS and with some corneal disorders experience pain. Pain associated with corneal disease is often described as a foreign sensation, whereas in OIS there is usually a deep eye or brow ache. Similar to the transient visual loss, the pain associated with OIS is more prominent when the patient is upright and often relieved by lying down. A description of the visual loss may also be helpful in distinguishing these mechanisms. Patients with visual loss due to corneal disease typically describe seeing halos, monocular diplopia and ghost images, whereas in OIS vision is dim and sometimes "blotchy".

In the above case, visual disturbance due to corneal dystrophy produced sufficient fluctuation to suggest a vascular disorder. The stereotypic timing of visual loss associated with awakening and the long duration of the attacks pointed to ocular disease as the cause.

Diagnosis: Transient monocular visual loss due to corneal decompensation

Tip: Transient visual loss due to ocular disease can usually be distinguished from retinal ischemic disease based just on the history.

FURTHER READING

Monocular diplopia

M. B. Bender, Polyopia and monocular diplopia of cerebral origin. *Arch Neurol Psychiatr*, **323** (1945), 38.

K. C. Golnik, E. Eggenberger, Symptomatic corneal topographic change induced by reading in downgaze. *J Neuroophthalmol*, **21** (2001), 199–204.

J. D. Trobe. *The Neurology of Vision*. Oxford: Oxford Press, 2001.

Hypertensive retinopathy

J. D. M. Gass. *Stereoscopic Atlas of Macular Diseases*, 4th edn. St. Louis: Mosby, 1997.

S. S. Hayreh, G. E. Servais, P. S. Virdi *et al.*, Fundus lesions in malignant hypertension. III. Arterial blood pressure, biochemical and fundus changes. *Ophthalmology*, **92** (1985), 45–59.

V. H. Lee, E. F. M. Wijdicks, E. M. Manno, A. A. Rubinstein, Clinical spectrum of reversible posterior leukoencephalopathy syndrome. *Arch Neurol*, **65** (2008), 205–10.

Twinkling scotoma

W. A. Fletcher, R. K. Imes, D. Goodman, W. F. Hoyt, Acute idiopathic blind spot enlargement: a big blind spot syndrome without disc edema. *Arch Ophthalmol*, **106** (1988), 44–9.

D. J. Gass, A. Agarwal, I. U. Scott, Acute zonal occult outer retinopathy: a long-term follow-up study. *Am J Ophthalmol*, **134** (2002), 329–39.

G. T. Liu, N. J. Schatz, S. L. Galetta *et al.*, Persistent positive visual phenomena in migraine. *Neurology*, **45** (1995), 664–8.

C. P. Panayiotopoulos, Elementary visual hallucinations in migraine and epilepsy. *J Neurol Neurosurg Psychiatry*, **57** (1994), 1371–4.

Central retinal artery occlusion

V. Biousse, O. Calvetti, B. Bruce, N. J. Newman, Thrombolysis for central retinal artery occlusion. *J Neuroophthalmol*, **27** (2007), 215–30.

S. S. Hayreh, M. B. Zimmerman, Central retinal artery occlusion: visual outcome. *Am J Ophthalmol*, **140** (2005), 376–91.

D. Yuzurihara, H. Iijima, Visual outcome in central and branch retinal artery occlusion. *Jpn J Ophthalmol*, **48** (2004), 490–2.

Hypovitaminosis A

N. J. Newman, A. Capone, H. F. Leeper *et al.*, Clinical and subclinical ophthalmic findings with retinol deficiency. *Ophthalmology*, **101** (1994), 1077–83.

V. Purvin, M. L. Slavin, Through a shade darkly. *Surv Ophthalmol*, **43** (1999), 335–40.

Cancer-associated retinopathy

L. Bataller, J. Dalmau, Neuro-ophthalmology and paraneoplastic syndromes. *Curr Opin Neurol*, **17** (2004), 3–8.

D. M. Jacobson, H. D. Pomeranz, Paraneoplastic diseases of neuro-ophthalmic interest. In N. R. Miller, N. J. Newman, V. Biousse, J. B. Kerrison, eds., *Walsh and Hoyt's Clinical Neuro-Ophthalmology*, 6th edn. Philadelphia: Lippincott Williams and Wilkins, 2005, Vol. **2**, Chapter 36, pp. 1715–58.

R. A. Sawyer, J. B. Selhorst, L. E. Zimmerman, W. F. Hoyt, Blindness caused by photoreceptor degeneration as a remote effect of cancer. *Am J Ophthamol*, **81** (1976), 606–13.

Corneal decompensation

R. C. Arffa, *Grayson's Diseases of the Cornea*, 4th edn. St. Louis: Mosby, 1997.

Glaucoma

R. R. Allingham, K. F. Damji, S. Freedman *et al.*, Optic nerve, retina and choroid. In *Shields' Textbook of Glaucoma*, 5th edn. Philadelphia: Lippincott Williams and Wilkins, 2004, pp. 73–116.

M. E. Gilbert, D. Friedman, Migraine and anisocoria. *Surv Ophthalmol*, **52** (2007), 209–12.

J. B. Jonas, W. M. Budde, Diagnosis and pathogenesis of glaucomatous optic neuropathy: morphological aspects. *Progress Retina Eye Res*, **19** (2000), 1–40.

R. Nesher, E. Epstein, Y. Stern, E. Assia, G. Nesher, Headaches as the main presenting symptom of subacute angle closure glaucoma. *Headache*, **45** (2004), 172–6.

S. D. Piette, R. C. Sergott, Pathological optic-disc cupping. *Curr Opin Ophthalmol*, **17** (2006), 1–6.

J. D. Trobe, J. S. Glaser, J. Cassady, J. Herschler, D. R. Anderson, Nonglaucomatous excavation of the optic disc. *Arch Ophthalmol*, **98** (1980), 1046–50.

2

When orbital disease is mistaken for neurologic disease

In most patients with orbital disease, the clinical presentation includes signs and symptoms that help localize the disease process to the orbit. Typical features include eye pain or pressure, proptosis, periorbital swelling, eyelid abnormalities, conjunctival injection and chemosis. Difficulty recognizing that the disease localizes to the orbit may occur when these clinical manifestations are subtle or even absent. Mistakes in clinical localization may be further compounded by misinterpretation of radiographic studies, because imaging modalities designed to detect intracranial pathology are often inadequate for identifying orbital abnormalities.

In cases lacking obvious signs of orbital disease, there are usually other aspects of the history or examination that are helpful in localization; finding them may require a little additional effort and expertise. Eye pain in itself is non-localizing, but pain that increases with, or is provoked by, eye movement indicates an orbital rather than intracranial source. Diffuse conjunctival injection is readily appreciated but, when focal, may only be found by examining the globe in eccentric positions including manual elevation of the lid (Figures 2.1 and 2.2). Chemosis may be similarly focal.

Careful examination is also critical for detecting mild degrees of proptosis or enophthalmos. Changes in globe position are best detected by viewing the patient from above or below and observing globe position relative to the orbital rim (Figure 2.3). Making this judgement while seated directly in front of the patient is notoriously unreliable because our impression of globe position is always influenced by lid position. Thus, lid retraction will be mistakenly perceived as proptosis (Figure 2.4C), whereas a smaller palpebral fissure (as in Horner syndrome) will be perceived as enophthalmos.

Certain eyelid abnormalities help to localize the disease process to the orbit. The lower lids demonstrate large variations in normal position. While most lower lids strike the globe at the lower limbus, many individuals exhibit a significant degree of inferior scleral show as a normal variation (Figure 2.4). Others have lower lids that rest a few millimeters above the limbus. Upper lid position is generally more consistent among normal individuals. The normal upper lid rests approximately 2 mm below the limbus. By definition, visible sclera above the superior limbus indicates a retracted lid. The presence of lid retraction is usually pathologic and is most commonly due to thyroid eye disease.

In this chapter we deal with cases in which a primary complaint of diplopia, visual loss or pain occurred in the relative absence of typical manifestations of orbital disease, and was therefore mistakenly attributed to intracranial disease. In each case, specific aspects of the history or examination should have raised concern for orbital disease, and these features are highlighted.

Incidental elevation deficit

Case: A 40-year-old interior decorator was referred for neurologic consultation because of recurrent headaches for several years. She was generally in good health and had no focal neurologic symptoms.

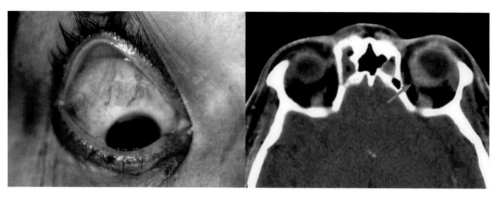

Figure 2.1 Marked hyperemia due to focal scleritis, only visible when the lid is manually elevated. Post-contrast CT of the same patient shows focal scleral enhancement posteriorly (arrow).

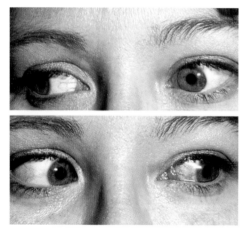

Figure 2.2 Young woman with orbital myositis. There is focal conjunctival injection over the left medial rectus insertion, best appreciated on eccentric gaze.

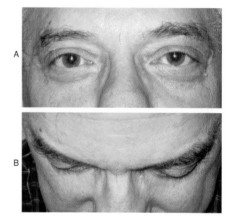

Figure 2.3 Examination technique for detecting proptosis. (A) Patient with mild left proptosis. The appearance of the globes seems normal when viewed face-to-face. (B) When viewed from above it is evident that the left globe is in fact proptotic relative to the right, protruding beyond the brow ridge.

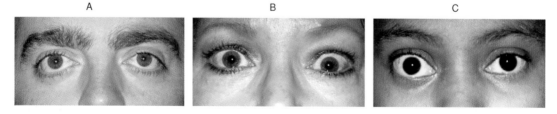

Figure 2.4 Normal and abnormal lid position. (A) A normal individual with prominent eyes due to shallow orbits, producing scleral show beneath the limbus bilaterally. (B) Bilateral upper lid retraction due to thyroid eye disease. Note superior scleral show. (C) Unilateral lid retraction in a young woman with asymmetric Graves' disease. The proptotic appearance of her right eye is an optical illusion due to lid retraction.

Physical examination was normal except for impairment of upgaze in the right eye. This was thought to represent a partial right third nerve palsy, and ancillary testing was therefore obtained. Brain MRI, CT of the orbits and a variety of blood tests were all normal or negative. A cerebral arteriogram was obtained to rule out an intracranial aneurysm, and results of this test were normal as well (see Chapter 10, Headache and third nerve palsy, for further discussion of imaging a suspected aneurysm).

She was referred for neuro-ophthalmic consultation. On examination, the eyes were aligned in primary position by cross-cover testing. Eye movements were full except for elevation of the right eye, which was limited, most prominently on gaze up and right (Figure 2.5). Saccadic velocity was normal in all directions, eyelid position and levator function were normal. Pupils were isocoric and briskly reactive to light.

What other mechanism could account for this patient's abnormal ocular motility besides a third nerve palsy?

Limitation of elevation can occur from myopathy, orbital restrictive disease, neuromuscular junction disease or supranuclear disorders of gaze. In this case, preservation of normal alignment in primary position suggests a restrictive mechanism. A similar pattern may also be seen in supranuclear gaze palsies such as internuclear ophthalmoplegia and supranuclear monocular upgaze palsy, but in such cases there is prominent slowing of saccades. If the marked degree of limited elevation in this patient's right eye were due to cranial nerve palsy, there would be a large angle right hypotropia in straight ahead gaze.

Review of her CT scan revealed an unrecognized blow-out fracture of the right orbital floor causing entrapment of the inferior rectus muscle (Figure 2.6). When these findings were reviewed with the patient, she recalled that at age eight she had fallen from a tree and struck her face, causing considerable bruising. At this point she realized that she had always had vague "blurring"

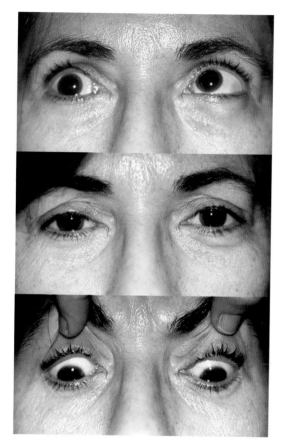

Figure 2.5 Ocular motility of a 40-year-old interior decorator with recurrent headaches. The eyes are normally aligned in primary position. Downgaze is full but elevation of the right eye is markedly limited, particularly in gaze up-right. (The pupils have been pharmacologically dilated.)

of vision on upgaze but had never sought medical attention for it. Difficulty recognizing that an ocular motility deficit is due to traumatic orbital disease may be particularly challenging in children in whom the traumatic event was unwitnessed. Ocular motility deficits may be present in the absence of external signs of trauma, sometimes termed a "white-eyed blowout". In this syndrome, a trapdoor orbital floor fracture incarcerates the inferior rectus, producing limitation of upgaze, as in the above patient.

A   B

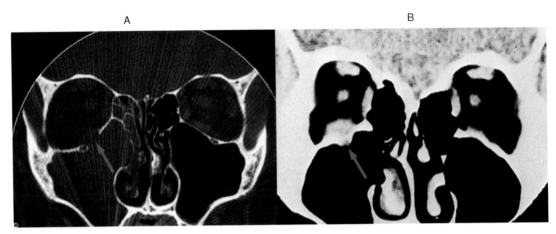

Figure 2.6 CT scan appearance of an orbital floor fracture. (A) Coronal image with bone-window settings in the above patient with limited elevation of the right eye reveals a discontinuity in the right orbital floor (arrow). (B) Soft tissue setting in a different patient with restrictive orbitopathy demonstrates entrapment of the inferior rectus muscle in the fracture (arrow).

Based on the above findings, this patient's motility disturbance was diagnosed as a long-standing muscle entrapment. As she was essentially asymptomatic, no specific treatment was indicated. Her headache pattern was consistent with migraine and was managed accordingly.

Discussion: The limited elevation of the right eye in this patient, particularly in gaze up and to the right, suggested weakness of the right superior rectus muscle, and extensive investigation was therefore undertaken for a presumed partial third nerve palsy. But her ocular motor problem was actually due to restriction of the inferior rectus muscle. Orbital restrictive disease, also termed *restrictive orbitopathy*, is characterized by loss of normal elasticity of an eye muscle, causing limited eye movement in a direction *opposite* to the action of the involved muscle (Figure 2.7). In this case, the inferior rectus muscle was entrapped in a long-standing but undiagnosed orbital floor fracture which caused tethering of the globe on attempted upgaze. In some cases of post-traumatic restrictive disease the muscle is not actually entrapped in the fracture but has lost elasticity due to scar-

ring. Graves' disease (thyroid eye disease) is another common cause of restrictive orbitopathy, often producing the same pattern seen here. Other less common forms include idiopathic orbital inflammation (orbital myositis), orbital tumors and iatrogenic events (e.g. inadvertent orbital penetration during sinus surgery).

Restrictive orbitopathy may involve one, several or all the extraocular muscles, and thus the pattern and magnitude of ophthalmoplegia depend on the muscles affected. Restrictive orbitopathy often mimics a neurologic ocular motor disorder; for example, a restricted medial rectus muscle produces an abduction deficit that simulates a sixth nerve palsy (Figure 2.8). In such cases, it is usually possible to distinguish between cranial neuropathy and orbital restrictive disease on clinical grounds without depending on neuro-imaging to identify the pathology.

Preserved alignment in primary position is not an invariable feature of restrictive orbitopathy but when present it is a very helpful finding. Normal saccadic velocity is another clue favoring restrictive orbital disease. Limitation of eye movement due to cranial nerve palsy or supranuclear disorders is

A   B

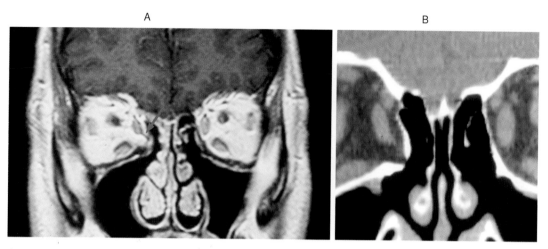

Figure 2.7 Another example of restrictive orbitopathy following trauma. This patient appeared to have a right sixth nerve palsy following head injury. (A) Coronal T1-weighted non-contrast MRI shows a thin band of tissue tethering the medial rectus in an undiagnosed medial wall fracture. (B) Coronal CT also shows distortion of the medial rectus and better demonstrates the bony discontinuity.

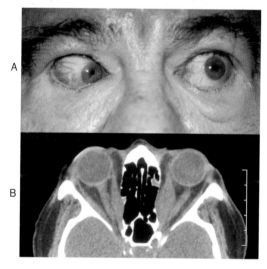

Figure 2.8 Restrictive orbitopathy due to thyroid eye disease. (A) There is incomplete abduction of the left eye, suggesting a left sixth nerve palsy and a right hypotropia. Bilateral lid retraction and conjunctival injection suggest the correct diagnosis of Graves' disease. (B) Axial non-contrast orbital CT shows fusiform enlargement of the medial rectus muscles, left greater than right.

typically accompanied by slowing of saccadic velocity. In contrast, the two conditions in which normal saccadic velocity is preserved despite eye movement limitation are *restrictive orbitopathy* and *myasthenia.* This differential feature is less helpful in cases with only minimal limitation of eye movement, in which slowing of saccadic velocity may be difficult to detect without the aid of recording devices.

The fact that only one eye muscle was involved in the above case was an additional helpful feature. If this patient's ocular motor dysfunction were due to a third nerve palsy, it would be a partial one. While partial third nerve palsies are common, isolated weakness of just one extraocular muscle is an extremely unusual presentation. Thus, it is important to consider other diagnostic possibilities when only one eye muscle is paretic, including myasthenia, internuclear ophthalmoplegia, myopathy and orbital restrictive disease.

Diagnosis: Orbital floor fracture with muscle entrapment

Tip: Restrictive orbitopathy can mimic neurologic ocular motor disorders. Normal ocular alignment

A

B

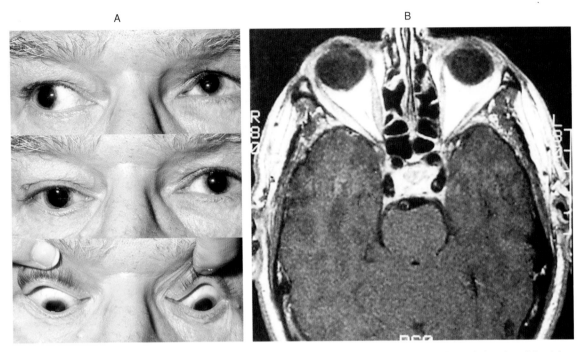

Figure 2.9 A 62-year-old man with chronic painless vertical diplopia. (A) There is markedly limited elevation of the right eye when abducted. Depression is full and the eyes are aligned on downgaze. (The pupils have been pharmacologically dilated.) (B) Axial contrast-enhanced T1-weighted MRI of the head shows no cause for his diplopia.

in primary position and normal saccadic velocity in the direction of paresis should suggest restrictive orbitopathy, even in the absence of typical orbital signs and symptoms.

Painless vertical diplopia

Case: This 62-year-old engineer had a one-year history of painless vertical diplopia that remained undiagnosed despite a variety of neurodiagnostic tests. After some initial progression he felt that his double vision had remained stable. His medical history was unremarkable except for well-controlled hypertension. Neuro-ophthalmic examination showed a 30-diopter left hypertropia in primary position with limitation of right eye elevation that was most marked with the eye abducted (Figure 2.9A). Infraduction was full and saccadic velocities were normal, as was the remainder of the

examination. A CBC, ESR, acetylcholine-receptor antibody titers and thyroid function tests were normal, as was a brain MRI (Figure 2.9B).

What clinical features help to localize the source of this patient's ocular motility disorder?

The normal saccadic velocity in the face of marked limitation of eye movement speaks strongly against supranuclear or cranial nerve dysfunction and points instead to either myasthenia or orbital restrictive disease (see Chapter 7, Farmer with an adduction deficit). The absence of variability over a one-year time period would be unusual for myasthenia. This pattern of motility disturbance (decreased elevation with the eye abducted) is typical of orbital restrictive disease, specifically due to loss of inferior rectus muscle elasticity. This is the most frequently affected extraocular

A   B

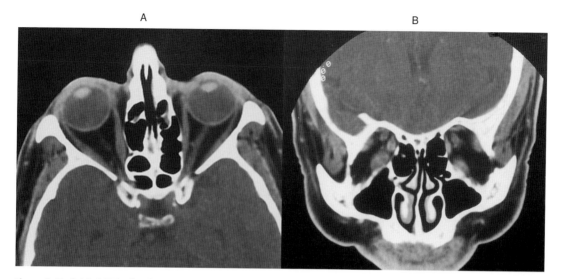

Figure 2.10 Orbital CT in the above patient with vertical diplopia. (A) The axial contrast-enhanced image is nearly normal, showing just subtle thickening of the right medial rectus muscle. In retrospect, this abnormality of the medial rectus could also be seen on the MRI. (B) The coronal image is much more helpful, demonstrating enlargement of the right inferior rectus muscle.

muscle in patients with thyroid eye disease, and therefore this pattern of motility disturbance is characteristic.

Based on the examination features described above, a dedicated CT scan of the orbits was obtained. This study showed a slightly plumper right medial rectus muscle compared to the left medial rectus and definite enlargement of the right inferior rectus muscle consistent with thyroid eye disease (Figure 2.10).

Discussion: This case illustrates an important point regarding the radiographic diagnosis of orbital disease. While brain MRI may detect orbital pathology in some patients, in other cases important findings will be missed if dedicated orbit views are not obtained. This is particularly true for abnormalities of the vertical eye muscles, as illustrated by this case. The horizontal rectus muscles are well visualized with axial views, which are often included in standard head scans, but coronal sections are needed to adequately evaluate the vertical muscles.

MRI is often considered preferable to CT because of its higher spatial resolution and superior soft tissue detail. Indeed, MRI is more sensitive than CT for inflammatory orbital disorders such as scleritis, optic neuritis and optic perineuritis (see below, Painful optic neuropathy) and is also superior for the detection of disease within the optic canal. However, CT scanning is a good alternative for demonstrating most orbital pathology and may be preferable in certain settings. CT provides excellent visualization of disorders of the extraocular muscles, such as thyroid eye disease. CT is preferable for all cases of trauma, for evaluating changes in the orbital bones and for demonstrating calcification, as in optic nerve sheath meningiomas and optic disc drusen. Whether MRI or CT is used, adequate orbital imaging includes both axial and coronal views.

This case also illustrates the limitations of thyroid function tests for the determination of Graves' orbitopathy. Abnormal test results (e.g. elevated T4 levels and suppressed TSH or, occasionally, low thyroid levels and elevated TSH) are helpful when present but are not required for the diagnosis, which remains a clinical one.

Diagnosis: Euthyroid Graves' disease

Tip: Orbital disease may be missed if dedicated orbit views are not obtained. Vertical muscle imbalance is best investigated with coronal views.

Fatigable ptosis

Case: A 58-year-old engineer noted drooping of his right upper eyelid that was minimal upon awakening each morning but worsened when he was tired (Figure 2.11). His past ocular history was positive only for bilateral cataract extraction two years earlier. He denied diplopia, dysphagia, hoarseness and limb weakness. Based on his description of variable ptosis, myasthenia gravis was suspected.

How is lid fatigability objectively demonstrated?

"Fatigable ptosis" refers to the demonstration of weakness of the levator that increases with prolonged use of the muscle and is a classic sign of myasthenia. To elicit this sign, the patient is asked to look up, with a minimal amount of blinking, for at least one minute. A lid that is weak from neuromuscular junction disease descends to a ptotic position, whereas a normal lid is able to maintain an extreme upward position. Attempts to elicit this finding by having the patient make repeated up and down excursions are unlikely to effectively demonstrate fatigability because the levator can recover each time the eye is in downgaze.

Another method for demonstrating myasthenic fatigability is termed *Cogan's lid twitch*. This sign is elicited by asking the patient to look down for 10–15 seconds then rapidly redirect gaze to primary position. In the downgaze position, the levator muscle is actively inhibited, allowing the neuromuscular junction a period of rest. Upon returning to primary position there is a brief overshoot of the myasthenic lid, followed by a resettling to its original ptotic position. In addition to Cogan's sign, myas-

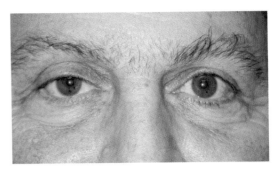

Figure 2.11 External appearance of a 58-year-old engineer with variable right upper lid ptosis. In addition to the lower position of the right upper lid, the superior lid crease is higher on that side.

thenic lids often demonstrate small spontaneous twitches due to variable neuromuscular blockade.

Some patients with myasthenia also have weakness of the orbicularis oculi muscles. This is an extremely helpful finding when present, because it indicates *myopathic* lid weakness. The important point here is that the levator and orbicularis muscles are innervated by different cranial nerves (the levator being supplied by the third nerve and the orbicularis by the seventh) and therefore the presence of weakness that involves both eyelid opening and closing effectively rules out a third nerve palsy as the cause of ptosis.

What other forms of ptosis might share a similar history of worsening with sustained use?

Any type of acquired ptosis may have a fatigable quality. In particular, individuals with *aponeurotic ptosis*, which represents a disinsertion of the levator aponeurosis from the tarsal plate, often report worsening ptosis later in the day and when relaxed, as in reading. Horner syndrome, in which there is sympathetic denervation of the tarsal muscles, may also cause mild ptosis which can vary depending on the degree of the patient's volitional use of the intact levator palpebrae muscle.

On examination, this patient's ocular motility and pupillary function were normal. There was no demonstrable fatigability of the levator muscle and

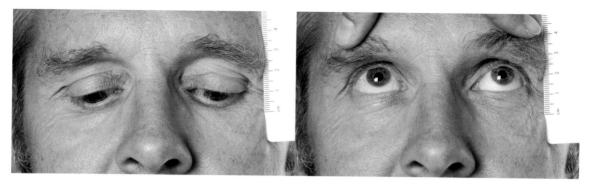

Figure 2.12 Technique for measuring levator function. The patient is first asked to look down, then up. The full excursion of the upper lid margin is measured. Note that frontalis action is minimized by manual pressure on the brow.

he did not show any of the above myasthenic lid findings. The superior lid crease was noted to be higher and deeper on the right side, a finding associated with dehiscence of the levator aponeurosis from the tarsal plate. Levator function, measured as the excursion of the upper lid from extreme downgaze to extreme upgaze, was 13 mm in both eyes (normal range 12–17 mm). Based on these findings, a diagnosis of aponeurotic ptosis was made. He was not sufficiently troubled by his ptosis to embark on surgery and he was therefore followed conservatively without a change in his ptosis over several years.

Discussion: The muscle that is primarily responsible for raising the eyelid is the levator palpebrae superioris. The levator muscle originates at the orbital apex and travels anteriorly along the orbital roof. Just behind the orbital rim, the muscle transitions into a broad tendon, termed the levator aponeurosis, which spreads out like a fan and curves down to insert into the tarsal plate of the lid. This insertion point is the anatomic basis for the eyelid crease. The sympathetically innervated superior tarsal muscle (Müller's muscle) lies under the levator aponeurosis and acts as an accessory muscle. It typically contributes 2 mm to the resting height of the lid.

Acquired ptosis can be classified as myogenic, neurogenic or aponeurotic. The most common form is *aponeurotic ptosis*, which is caused by thin-

ning and disinsertion of the aponeurosis. The most important risk factor for aponeurotic dehiscence is advancing age, leading some to refer to it as *"senile ptosis".* Other factors, however, can precipitate levator dehiscence, including stretching of the lid during intraocular surgery, chronic rubbing of the eyes or long-term use of contact lenses. A higher lid crease on the side of the ptosis and a deepening of the superior lid sulcus are suggestive of aponeurotic ptosis.

The key diagnostic feature in ptosis due to levator dehiscence is preservation of levator function. Because the function of the levator muscle is still intact, the extent of lid excursion remains normal even though the muscle has assumed a new (lower) position. In contrast, levator function is decreased in neurogenic and myopathic ptosis. Levator function is easily measured in millimeters as the vertical distance that the lid travels from extreme downgaze to extreme upgaze (Figure 2.12). Normal levator function is 12 to 17 mm and is symmetric between the two eyes.

A second helpful examination feature for distinguishing aponeurotic from neurogenic or myogenic ptosis is the position of the eyelid crease. In disinsertion, the aponeurosis is dragged superiorly and drags the eyelid crease with it. Thus, in aponeurotic ptosis there is typically elevation of the eyelid crease, shortening the distance to the brow. This elevation is not a feature of other forms of ptosis.

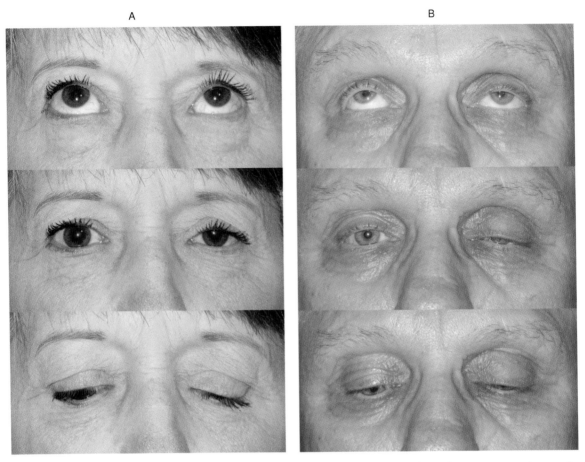

Figure 2.13 Levator dehiscence vs. neurogenic ptosis. (A) Left upper lid ptosis secondary to long-term contact lens use. In primary gaze the left lid is lower than the right. In downgaze, the asymmetry of lid position between the two eyes is the same as in primary gaze. Notice that the full excursion of the left lid is equal to that of the right. (B) Left upper lid ptosis secondary to partial third NP. Notice that upper lid position is similar in the two eyes on downgaze despite marked left upper lid ptosis in primary gaze. Excursion of the left upper lid is decreased compared to the right.

A third observation that is often helpful is a comparison of lid position in upgaze, primary position and downgaze. In aponeurotic dehiscence, the ptotic lid is lower than the normal lid not only in primary position but also in downgaze (Figure 2.13). In contrast, in myopathic or neuropathic ptosis the lid position is normal on downgaze.

Although drooping of the lids that is worse later in the day is commonly reported by patients with myasthenia, it is not specific and may occur in other forms of acquired ptosis. Most individuals can overcome ptosis to some extent by various means, including overaction of the frontalis muscles, increased effort directed to the levator muscles (thereby increasing the firing rate) and by assuming a chin-up head position. This extra effort, however, is difficult to sustain, and so ptosis often worsens with fatigue. Thus, patients with ptosis of any mechanism often report that their droopy lid is worse later in the day and when they are tired.

Diagnosis: Levator dehiscence

Tip: In a patient with ptosis, normal levator function implies aponeurotic ptosis, whereas subnormal levator function indicates neurogenic or myogenic ptosis.

Painful ptosis and diplopia

Case: A 48-year-old healthy secretary developed severe pain over the left brow accompanied by vertical diplopia. Examination revealed mild left upper lid ptosis, left hypotropia and limited elevation of the left eye (Figure 2.14). The remainder of her ophthalmic and neurologic examination was normal. She received a diagnosis of superior division palsy, a distinctive pattern of partial third nerve palsy in which weakness is limited to the superior rectus and

levator muscles. A brain MRI with attention to the cavernous sinus showed no cause for third nerve palsy and a lumbar puncture was also normal.

What is the anatomic significance of a superior division palsy?

The third nerve exits the midbrain and passes anteriorly through the subarachnoid cistern where it lies in close proximity to a number of vascular structures. The nerve then pierces the dura near the top of the clivus to enter the cavernous sinus. Just before entering the orbit via the superior orbital fissure, the third nerve splits into two divisions: a *superior division* containing motor fibers to the superior rectus and levator, and an *inferior division* containing the remaining motor fibers plus the parasympathetic fibers to the iris sphincter and ciliary body. Based on this anatomy, a divisional third nerve palsy should localize to the anterior cavernous

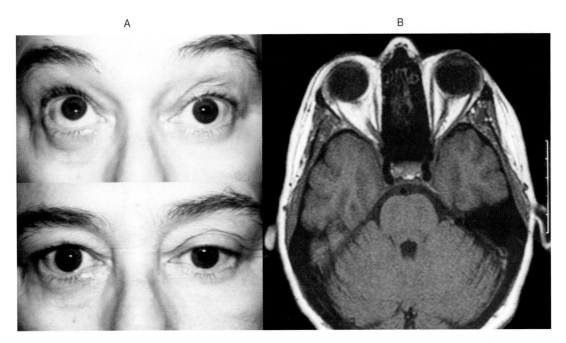

A B

Figure 2.14 A 48-year-old woman with apparent superior division third nerve palsy. (A) In primary position there is moderate left upper lid ptosis and hypotropia. The pupils are isocoric. On upgaze there is incomplete elevation of the left eye. (B) Axial non-contrast T1-weighted brain MRI shows an incidental left arachnoid cyst but is otherwise normal.

sinus or superior orbital fissure where the nerve splits. There are, however, well-documented cases in which a divisional palsy was caused by a lesion more proximal in the course of the nerve, indicating that this topographic division occurs earlier in its course. Nevertheless, when imaging a patient with a superior division palsy, attention should be directed initially to the anterior cavernous sinus and superior orbital fissure. If no abnormality is found, the scope of the radiographic investigation should be enlarged to ensure that the rest of the third nerve pathway has been adequately imaged.

The investigation thus far has revealed no intracranial pathology. How would you proceed?

Further questioning revealed that the patient's pain was decidedly worse with eye movement, particularly on upgaze. Based on this additional history, orbital disease was suspected and a dedicated orbital MRI was obtained, which showed abnormal enhancement and enlargement of the left superior rectus/levator complex (Figure 2.15). Evaluation for inflammatory, infectious, granulomatous and neoplastic etiologies was unrevealing. She was diagnosed with *orbital myositis*, a localized form of idiopathic orbital inflammatory syndrome, and treated with oral prednisone. Within two days she experienced complete relief of pain, and by one week later her diplopia had resolved completely. The patient was weaned off steroids over the next eight weeks, and she has had no recurrence in six years.

Discussion*: Idiopathic orbital inflammatory disease*, also referred to as *orbital pseudotumor*, is a non-granulomatous inflammation of orbital structures with no known local or systemic causes. It may arise in any age group, though most commonly affects young and middle aged adults. Clinical manifestations vary according to the location, severity and duration of the inflammatory process, and clinical subtypes can be defined by the predominant

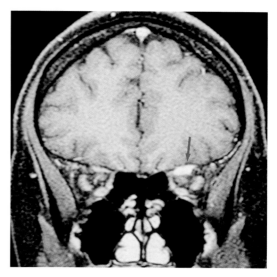

Figure 2.15 Orbital MRI of the above patient. A coronal post-contrast, fat-suppressed T1-weighted image through the mid-orbit shows enlargement and enhancement of the superior rectus/levator muscle complex on the left side (arrow).

site of involvement. These include dacryoadenitis (lacrimal gland), myositis (one or more extraocular muscles), scleritis, optic perineuritis, mass-like lesions at the orbital apex and diffuse infiltrative inflammation.

Pain is the most common feature of idiopathic orbital inflammation and is the symptom that usually prompts patients to seek medical attention. Those with extraocular muscle involvement also experience diplopia. Accompanying signs of orbitopathy such as periorbital edema, lid swelling, conjunctival injection, proptosis and chemosis are present in most patients. In the patient under discussion, myositis was limited to the superior rectus/levator complex. Because of the very focal nature of the inflammation in this case, typical orbital findings were absent, thus leading to the mistaken impression of a partial third nerve palsy due to intracranial disease. Pain in orbital inflammatory disease can be quite severe and is typically exacerbated by eye movement. This feature is particularly helpful for directing attention to the orbit

A

B

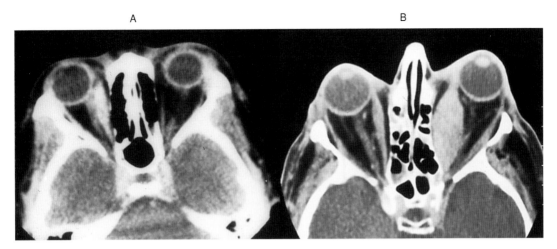

Figure 2.16 Extraocular muscle appearance in orbital myositis vs. Graves' disease. (A) Axial post-contrast CT in a patient with orbital myositis demonstrates intense enhancement and tubular enlargement of the right medial rectus muscle extending anteriorly to involve the tendinous insertion. (B) In a patient with Graves' orbitopathy the CT shows diffuse spindle-shaped enlargement of the left medial rectus muscle with sparing of the tendon.

as the site of the disease process. Some intracranial processes, such as meningitis, can be associated with pain on eye movement, but in such cases the pain is usually bilateral and accompanied by headache.

The diagnosis of orbital inflammatory disease is usually based on a combination of the clinical and neuro-imaging findings. A post-contrast MRI with coronal views and fat suppression is the preferred study, but in many cases a post-contrast orbit CT can suffice as well since the key findings are essentially the same on both. In orbital myositis, the chief finding is enlargement of one or more extraocular muscles. The tendons are frequently thickened, leading to a tubular configuration of muscle enlargement which is in contrast to the spindle-shaped muscle enlargement characteristic of Graves' orbitopathy (Figure 2.16). In some patients with orbital pseudotumor, there is also streaky enhancement of the orbital fat or enlargement of the lacrimal gland, and these findings are helpful for confirming the diagnosis. While these differences are helpful for distinguishing these two entities radiographically, the typical clinical presentation of orbital pseudotumor with acute pain is so

different from the insidious, non-painful presentation of Graves' disease that the two disorders are readily distinguished on clinical grounds in most cases.

Idiopathic orbital inflammatory syndrome is a diagnosis of exclusion, requiring a thorough evaluation for systemic inflammatory disorders (Table 2.1). A biopsy is not considered necessary for the diagnosis if the history, radiographic findings and response to steroids fit the disease profile. Biopsy is reserved for patients with atypical clinical findings, lack of steroid responsiveness, persistent radiographic abnormality despite treatment and in some cases with recurrence following treatment.

Occasional patients with mild forms of idiopathic orbital inflammation can be managed with non-steroidal anti-inflammatory agents, but in most cases corticosteroids are the mainstay of treatment. Oral (as opposed to intravenous) steroids are usually sufficient and the response is typically dramatic, particularly the resolution of pain within 24–48 hours. Most patients respond well to oral prednisone 60–100 mg daily for two weeks with a slow taper thereafter. Despite this positive initial

Table 2.1 Etiologies of orbital inflammatory disease

Sarcoidosis
Syphilis
Cysticercosis
Lyme disease
Whipple's disease
Herpes zoster
Inflammatory bowel disease
Wegener's granulomatosis
Systemic lupus erythematosus
Rheumatoid arthritis
Scleroderma
Psoriatic arthropathy
Giant cell myocarditis
Kawasaki disease

response, about half of patients experience a later recurrence of orbital inflammation.

Diagnosis: Idiopathic orbital myositis

Tip: Orbital inflammation involving the superior rectus and levator muscles can mimic a superior division third nerve palsy. The presence of pain that is exacerbated by eye movement points to an orbital rather than intracranial process.

Painful optic neuropathy

Case: A 24-year-old waitress developed mild blurring of vision in the left eye associated with moderately severe periocular pain that was worse with eye movement. Three weeks after onset of symptoms, visual acuity was 20/20 in each eye and color vision was normal but there was a trace relative afferent pupillary defect (RAPD) on the left side. The right optic disc was normal, the left disc was mildly swollen. A brain MRI was normal. She received a presumptive diagnosis of idiopathic optic neuritis and was managed expectantly.

Her eye pain persisted and vision worsened further. On examination eight weeks after onset, her acuity had declined to 20/80 OS and she could identify only 5 of 15 color plates. There was now a

small but definite (1+) left RAPD. The left optic disc was still swollen and Goldmann perimetry demonstrated an inferior arcuate scotoma in the left eye (Figure 2.17). All findings in the right eye were normal.

Is this patient's clinical course consistent with a diagnosis of optic neuritis?

The natural history of optic neuritis includes stabilization of vision and improvement of pain within two weeks of onset. Resolution of disc edema, if present, usually occurs by four weeks after onset. In contrast, this patient still had pain and disc edema eight weeks after onset, and her evaluation showed further progression of visual loss between the third week and eighth week. In addition, the pattern of visual loss (arcuate defect rather than central loss) would be unusual for demyelinating optic neuritis.

What specific feature of her clinical course raises the possibility of orbital disease?

Pain with eye movement that is *severe and persistent* is atypical for demyelinating optic neuritis and more suggestive of orbital inflammatory disease. An MRI of the orbits with contrast enhancement and fat suppression was obtained and showed enhancement *around* the left intraorbital optic nerve, indicating inflammation of the optic nerve sheath rather than the nerve itself (Figure 2.18). Blood tests for systemic inflammatory disorders were all normal or negative and a diagnosis of idiopathic optic perineuritis was made. She was treated with 80 mg of prednisone per day and experienced dramatic improvement of vision and complete resolution of pain. Her steroid dose was tapered over the next few months and she continued to do well.

Discussion: Inflammation involving the optic nerve *sheath* is termed *optic perineuritis* (OPN) and is considered a variant of idiopathic orbital inflammatory syndrome (described in the preceding case). Occasional cases of optic perineuritis are

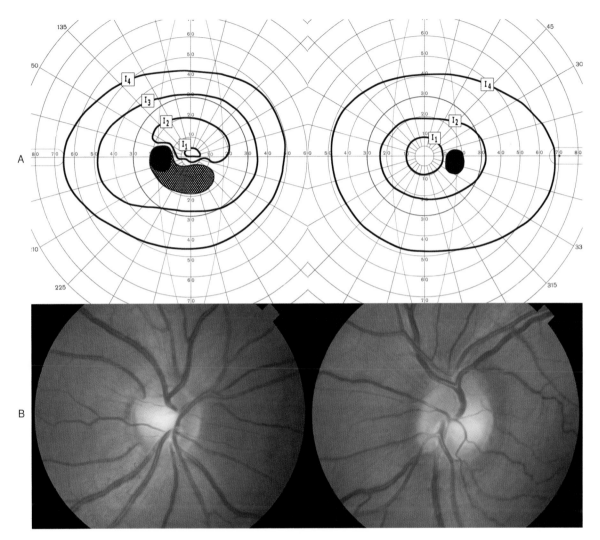

Figure 2.17 Examination findings in a 24-year-old waitress with painful visual loss in the left eye. (A) Goldmann perimetry shows an inferior arcuate scotoma in the left eye. (B) The right disc is normal, the left disc is mildly swollen.

due to a specific systemic inflammatory disorder such as sarcoidosis, Wegener's granulomatosis, giant cell arteritis or syphilis (see Table 2.1 above), but in most cases inflammation is isolated to the orbit, and idiopathic. Although OPN shares some similarities with demyelinating optic neuritis, there are several clinical differences which are helpful for distinguishing between these two disorders (Table 2.2).

Similar to optic neuritis, idiopathic OPN affects women more often than men. The age range, however, is different: optic neuritis usually occurs in young adults whereas the age range in OPN is broader. Optic neuritis typically causes decreased visual acuity whereas in patients with OPN acuity is often spared. The natural history of these two disorders also differs. In contrast to the self-limited nature of optic neuritis, pain and visual loss in OPN

Table 2.2 Optic neuritis vs. optic perineuritis: clinical features

	Optic Neuritis	Optic Perineuritis
Age at onset	Usually young adults, only 15% >50 yrs	Broader range, about 40% >50 yrs
Visual loss	Usually central	Often paracentral/arcuate
Time course	Progression over days	Progression over weeks
Natural history	Spontaneous recovery	Progressive visual loss
Response to steroid treatment	Variable	Prompt, dramatic
	Uncommon relapse after stopping	Relapse common after brief treatment
	Optic nerve enhancement	Peri-neural enhancement
	± white matter lesions	"Streaky" fat ± eye muscle enhancement

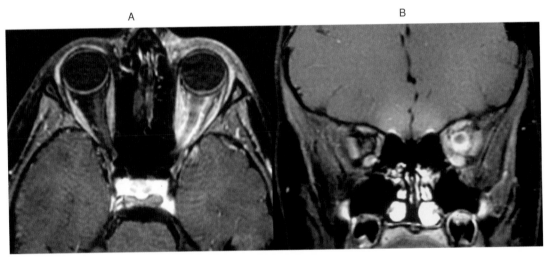

Figure 2.18 Fat-saturated T1-weighted post-contrast MRI in the above patient with idiopathic optic perineuritis. There is intense enhancement around the left optic nerve on (A) axial and (B) coronal views. There is also abnormal enhancement of the orbital fat and subtle enlargement of the inferior rectus muscle.

continue to progress. Unlike optic neuritis, patients with OPN show a dramatic response to steroids including a tendency to recur if steroids are discontinued too quickly.

The diagnosis of OPN is based on the radiographic (or occasionally histopathologic) findings. The characteristic picture is seen best on coronal post-contrast fat-suppressed MR images of the orbits, in which the inflammation of the optic nerve sheath appears as a bright doughnut of enhancement around the optic nerve. This radiographic appearance resembles that of optic nerve sheath meningioma, but the presence of pain and acute visual loss in OPN contrasts with the insidious and usually painless presentation in patients with meningioma.

The importance of distinguishing OPN from optic neuritis concerns both treatment and prognosis. In terms of visual outcome, steroid treatment is considered optional for patients with optic neuritis whereas, without treatment, patients with OPN experience continued pain and progressive visual loss. Patients with optic neuritis are at risk for the future development of multiple sclerosis whereas those with idiopathic OPN are more likely to experience a subsequent episode of recurrent painful visual loss but harbor no increased risk for systemic disease.

Diagnosis: Idiopathic optic perineuritis

Tip: Severe and persistent pain is atypical for optic neuritis and should suggest the possibility of optic perineuritis.

FURTHER READING

Orbital examination and restrictive orbitopathy

J. A. Garrity, R. S. Bahn, Pathogenesis of Graves' ophthalmopathy: implications for prediction, prevention and treatment. *Am J Ophthamol*, **142** (2007), 147–53.

J. A. Nerad. *Oculoplastic Surgery*. Philadelphia: Elsevier, 2001.

J. Rootman. *Diseases of the Orbit*, 2nd edn. Baltimore: Lippincott Williams and Wilkins, 2002.

Levator dehiscence

D. G. Cogan, Myasthenia gravis. A review of the disease and a description of lid twitch as a characteristic sign. *Arch Ophthalmol*, **74** (1965), 217–21.

R. C. Kersten, C. de Conciliis, D. R. Kulwin, Acquired ptosis in the young and middle-aged adult population. *Ophthalmology*, **102** (1995), 924–8.

Painful ptosis and diplopia

D. Jacobs, S. Galetta, Diagnosis and management of orbital pseudotumor. *Curr Opin Ophthalmol*, **13** (2002), 347–51.

S. M. Ksiazek, M. X. Repka, A. Maguire *et al.*, Divisional oculomotor nerve paresis caused by intrinsic brainstem disease. *Ann Neurol*, **26** (1989), 714.

B. Lacey, W. Chang, J. Rootman, Nonthyroid causes of extraocular muscle disease. *Surv Ophthalmol*, **44** (2000), 187–213.

S. J. A. Yuen, P. Rubin, Idiopathic orbital inflammation. Distribution, clinical features and treatment outcome. *Arch Ophthalmol*, **121** (2003), 491–9.

Optic perineuritis

J. J. Dutton, R. L. Anderson, Idiopathic inflammatory perioptic neuritis simulating optic nerve sheath meningioma. *Am J Ophthalmol*, **100** (1985), 424–30.

A. M. Fay, S. A. Kane, M. Kazim, W. S. Millar, J. G. Odel, Magnetic resonance imaging of optic perineuritis. *J Neuroophthalmol*, **17** (1997), 247–9.

V. Purvin, A. Kawasaki, D. M. Jacobson, Optic perineuritis: clinical and radiographic features. *Arch Ophthalmol*, **119** (2001), 1299–306.

3

Mistaking congenital anomalies for acquired disease

Congenital anomalies comprise a spectrum of disorders of varying severity. When severe, such anomalies are readily appreciated at birth or in early infancy. Examples of neuro-ophthalmic anomalies that present early in life include congenital esotropia, ptosis and severe bilateral optic nerve hypoplasia. Milder forms may not be detected until adulthood and may come to medical attention in several ways. In some cases, patients are asymptomatic, and their congenital anomaly is detected only when the visual system is evaluated for another purpose. Examples of this include persistent myelinated nerve fiber layer, pigmented lesions of the optic disc and partial forms of optic nerve hypoplasia. In other cases, the patient does have symptoms that could be due to a condition that resembles a congenital anomaly. An example of this scenario is the patient who seeks medical attention because of headaches and is found to have pseudopapilledema. In still others, an abnormality that has been present since birth only becomes symptomatic in adult life. For example, many forms of ocular misalignment can be kept in check by binocular fusion, only to decompensate in midlife for a variety of reasons. The Chiari malformation, while clearly a congenital malformation, often remains asymptomatic throughout childhood but causes progressive neurologic deficits in adulthood. Similarly, aqueductal stenosis may decompensate after years of stability.

Recognition of the congenital nature of an abnormality is important because unnecessary testing and treatment can then be avoided. In most cases there are sufficient clinical clues to help make this determination.

Headaches and elevated discs

Case: A 15-year-old high-school student consulted her family physician because of headaches. She had had an occasional "sick headache" since age eight but these had become more frequent over the past year. Her headaches were accompanied by nausea and photosensitivity and were usually relieved by sleep. She was unaware of any factors that precipitated her headaches. She was otherwise healthy and her growth and development had been normal. She denied pulsatile tinnitus, transient obscurations of vision and diplopia. Her general examination was normal, but fundus examination revealed bilateral optic disc elevation. This finding prompted a brain MRI that was normal. A lumbar puncture was recommended but, at her mother's request, she was sent first for neuro-ophthalmic consultation.

Visual acuity was 20/20 in each eye with normal color vision, pupillary responses and ocular motility. Visual field testing was normal by Goldmann perimetry. Fundus examination showed moderate elevation of both optic discs without opacification of the nerve fiber layer or venous engorgement (Figure 3.1). Based on the optic disc appearance, pseudopapilledema due to buried drusen was suspected.

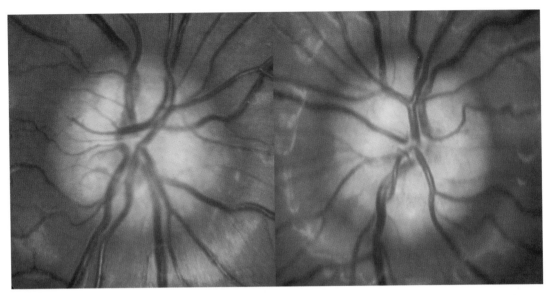

Figure 3.1 Fundus photographs in a 15-year-old girl with headaches. The optic discs are elevated, there is no central cup and the retinal veins have a normal caliber. Importantly, there is no opacification of the peri-papillary nerve fiber layer.

Is there a way to confirm the presence of drusen in this patient?

Drusen can be demonstrated with orbital ultra-sonography, CT scan or by demonstrating autofluor-escence. In this case, an orbital ultrasound (B-scan) was performed, which showed hyper-reflectivity within the disc substance of each eye, confirming a diagnosis of drusen (Figure 3.2). This patient's headaches were thought to be migrainous and were managed accordingly.

Discussion: Optic disc drusen are a common congenital anomaly, found in up to 2% of normal individuals. Drusen are inherited as an autosomal dominant trait but with irregular penetrance. Earlier theories held that individuals with drusen are born with a tendency to form small concretions within the optic disc, which may cause damage to optic nerve fibers either by direct compression or by interfering with blood supply. Current thinking, however, suggests that the initial step in the process of drusen formation involves leakage of axoplasmic material from neurons. Over time, this substance

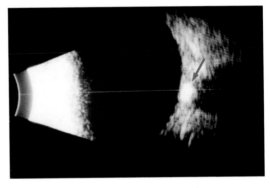

Figure 3.2 Orbital B-scan ultrasonogram shows hyper-reflectivity within the disc substance consistent with drusen (arrow).

tends to collect calcium, iron, mucopolysaccha-rides and other material (Figure 3.3). The reason for this axonal leakage is unclear, perhaps related to an anomaly of the lamina cribrosa rather than a metabolic defect of axoplasmic transport. Whatever the exact mechanism, we now view disc drusen as a form of chronic optic neuropathy that is very slowly progressive over a lifetime.

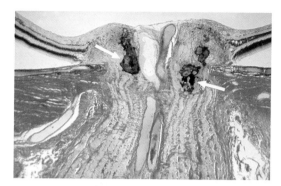

Figure 3.3 Cross section through the optic disc in an eye with buried drusen. Intrapapillary drusen appear as concretions within the substance of the prelaminar nerve head (arrows).

Disc drusen are bilateral in 75% of cases. The severity of drusen, both in terms of disc appearance and optic nerve function, is extremely variable. Visual field abnormalities are common, found in up to 87% of affected eyes. However, visual acuity is rarely reduced because the defects usually involve the arcuate or radial nerve fiber bundles rather than the papillomacular bundle. Occasionally, drusen are associated with vascular events involving the optic disc and retinal circulations, most notably anterior ischemic optic neuropathy and spontaneous hemorrhages into the nerve head. Such secondary complications can cause acute loss of vision that involves the central field and thus reduces visual acuity. Although drusen can produce slowly progressive visual loss over a lifetime, such deficits are not usually disabling. In most cases, the chief significance of drusen (and other forms of congenital disc elevation) is not that it *is* a serious condition, but rather that it *looks* like something serious, namely papilledema.

In young children, drusen are more likely to be buried, whereas in adults they are often visible on the disc surface (Figure 3.4). An effective technique for appreciating surface drusen is to use the smallest light of the direct ophthalmoscope to illuminate one part of the disc while observing another area. In this manner, light reflects off the side of small refractile bodies making them more apparent. Eyes

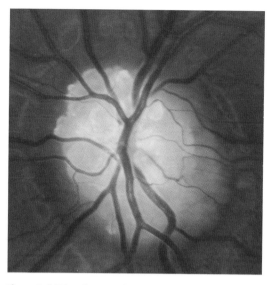

Figure 3.4 Disc photograph showing prominent drusen on the disc surface.

Table 3.1 Ophthalmoscopic features in papilledema vs. pseudopapilledema

Feature	Papilledema	Pseudopapilledema
Nerve fiber layer	Opacified	Normal (translucent)
Retinal veins	Dilated/non-pulsatile	Normal caliber ± pulsations
Capillary hyperemia	Yes	No
Retinal vasculature	Normal	Often anomalous
Physiologic cup	Fills in late	Usually absent
Hemorrhages	Nerve fiber layer	Deep crescentic
Peri-papillary pigment changes	No	Common

with buried drusen pose more of a diagnostic challenge, the specific task usually being the distinction between pseudopapilledema and papilledema (i.e. disc edema due to increased intracranial pressure). There are several ophthalmoscopic observations that are helpful for distinguishing between congenital and acquired disc elevation (see Table 3.1 – and Figures 3.5, 3.6 and 3.7). The most

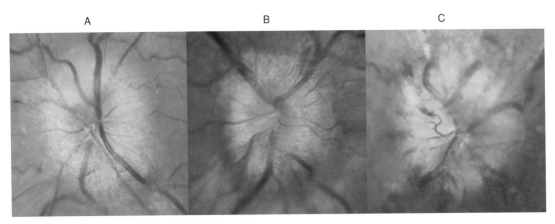

Figure 3.5 Fundus photographs of three different patients with increased intracranial pressure. (A) Papilledema in this case is mild, however still displays characteristic opacification of the nerve fiber layer, distinguishing this from pseudopapilledema. (B) More advanced disc edema with prominent capillary hyperemia and venous distention. (C) Severe papilledema with hemorrhages, exudates and obliteration of the physiologic cup.

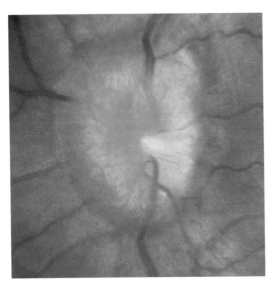

Figure 3.6 Papilledema. Despite well-developed disc swelling, there is preservation of a sharp disc margin, illustrating the limitation of using this feature to distinguish congenital from acquired disc elevation.

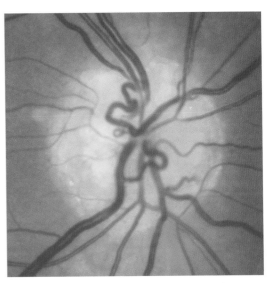

Figure 3.7 Optic disc drusen with anomalous branching of the retinal vasculature and prominent peri-papillary pigment changes, features that commonly accompany drusen.

sensitive and specific indicator of acquired disc edema is *opacification of the nerve fiber layer*. This opacification is best understood by recalling the pathophysiology of papilledema; namely obstruction or slowing of axoplasmic transport with resultant swelling of axons. Because the nerve fiber layer is between the examiner's eye and the patient's retinal blood vessels, such opacification is best appreciated by noting obscuration of these vessels (Figure 3.5A). The presence of "blurred

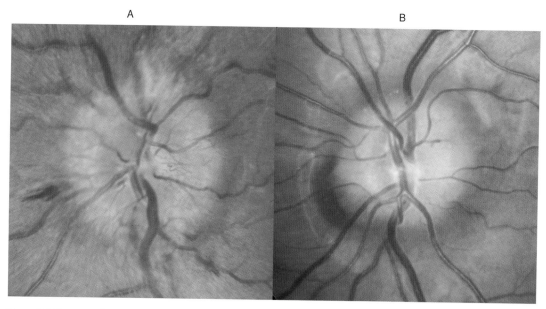

Figure 3.8 Patterns of optic disc hemorrhage. (A) In papilledema, hemorrhage is within the nerve fiber layer. (B) In contrast, in pseudopapilledema the hemorrhage is deep, within the peri-papillary retina, and has a typical crescentic shape.

disc margins" is *not* a particularly useful sign (Figure 3.6).

Examination of the retinal vessels can provide additional clues. In true papilledema, the capillaries on the disc surface are usually hyperemic and the retinal veins become tortuous, distended and non-pulsatile (Figure 3.5B). In addition, the branching pattern of the retinal vasculature is often anomalous in eyes with drusen (Figure 3.7). The absence of spontaneous pulsations is not a helpful differential finding since pulsations are visible in just 60% of the normal population; however their presence speaks strongly against increased ICP. Observing the size of the physiologic cup is also helpful. In most eyes with pseudopapilledema the cup is absent; in fact, the center of the disc is often the most elevated area. In contrast, filling in of the physiologic cup is a late event in the evolution of papilledema. In most cases, by the time the cup is obliterated, the nature of the disc elevation is no longer in question (Figure 3.5).

Disc hemorrhages may occur in either condition but the *pattern* of hemorrhage is informative. In papilledema, hemorrhages are typically within the nerve fiber layer (sometimes termed "flame" or "splinter" hemorrhages, Figure 3.8A) whereas in pseudopapilledema they are usually deep, are located just at the edge of the disc and have a crescentic shape (Figure 3.8B). Repeated hemorrhages of this sort lead to pigment alterations in the peri-papillary area, a common finding in eyes with drusen (Figure 3.7). In occasional cases, development of a subretinal neovascular net causes repeated hemorrhage and leakage into the surrounding retina.

Drusen can usually be suspected from the ophthalmoscopic appearance. Their presence can sometimes be confirmed on a non-contrast orbital CT, although with less sensitivity than ultrasound (Figure 3.9A). Drusen are not visible on MRI. In the hands of an experienced examiner, ultrasonography is the preferred investigative tool. Finding

A   B

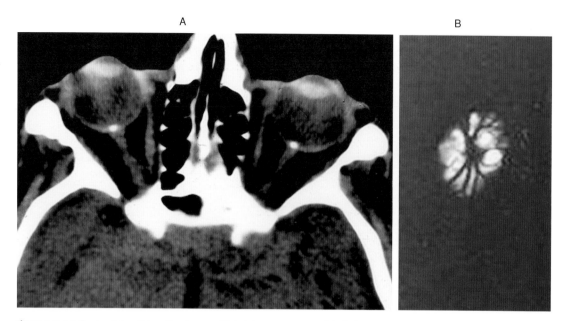

Figure 3.9 Methods of visualizing disc drusen. (A) Axial non-contrast orbit CT in a patient with bilateral drusen demonstrates calcification within each disc. (B) Intense autofluorescence in the patient whose disc is seen in Figure 3.4.

hyper-reflective signal within the substance of the optic disc confirms a diagnosis of buried drusen, whereas the presence of a widened nerve sheath is indirect evidence for increased intracranial pressure. Fundus photography also can be helpful: with the cobalt filter used for fluorescein angiography but without injection of dye, surface drusen may be revealed by their autofluorescence (Figure 3.9B). Fluorescein angiography can also furnish useful information: absence of leakage in the late phases of the study effectively rules out acquired disc edema.

In most cases, a diagnosis of pseudopapilledema can be established based on the history and examination findings, with particular emphasis on ophthalmoscopic findings. In some cases, the addition of ancillary testing, as described above, can be confirmatory. It is rarely necessary to proceed with a lumbar puncture to exclude causes of acquired disc edema. The diagnosis of congenitally anomalous discs should *not* be considered a diagnosis of exclusion.

Diagnosis: Buried drusen (pseudopapilledema)

Tip: Pseudopapilledema can usually be distinguished from acquired disc edema based on ophthalmoscopic appearance.

Inferior altitudinal visual field defects

Case: This 24-year-old receptionist was found to have an abnormal visual field on a routine screening test. The patient was unaware of the defect and had no visual or neurologic symptoms although she did acknowledge that she had always been considered clumsy and tended to trip over things. She was otherwise healthy. Family history was negative for neurologic or eye disease except for diabetic retinopathy in her mother. A more complete eye examination demonstrated visual acuity of 20/20 in each eye with normal color vision, pupillary responses and intraocular pressures. Goldmann perimetry confirmed an inferior altitudinal defect in each eye (Figure 3.10). The optic discs

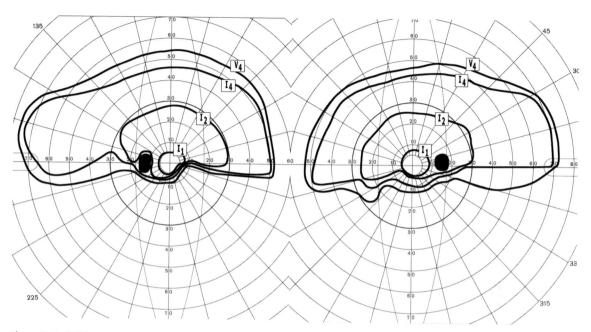

Figure 3.10 Goldmann perimetry demonstrates near-complete bilateral inferior altitudinal defects.

showed questionable pallor superiorly. Possible mechanisms that were considered for this patient's bilateral optic neuropathy included ischemia, compression, toxic injury and congenital anomaly.

Are there clues to the correct diagnosis in this case?

The diagnosis in this case can be deduced from two lines of evidence: the optic disc appearance and the family history. Careful inspection of the fundus reveals that the top of each optic disc is not actually pale but mal-developed (Figure 3.11). This disc appearance is diagnostic of a form of partial optic nerve hypoplasia that is found in the offspring of diabetic mothers. No additional testing was needed and the patient was reassured as to the benign and static nature of her congenital syndrome.

Discussion: Optic nerve hypoplasia is a congenital anomaly with a spectrum of clinical presentations. When severe and bilateral, the condition usually presents in infancy with poor fixation and nystag-

mus. The classic fundus picture is referred to as the "double-ring" or "halo" sign, in which a small optic disc is surrounded by a ring of bare sclera which usually is bordered by pigment (Figure 3.12). However, the appearance of optic disc hypoplasia is quite variable and the double-ring sign is found only in a minority of patients. In some cases, only a portion of the disc is hypoplastic, as in the above case, in which there is only half of a double-ring sign.

As in many congenital anomalies, the teratogenic insult is more time-specific than stimulus-specific. A variety of systemic events occurring at the six-week stage of embryogenesis have been associated with an increased risk of optic nerve hypoplasia (see Table 3.2). Optic nerve hypoplasia may occur as an isolated anomaly or may be associated with other abnormalities. The most common of these are absence of the septum pellucidum and agenesis of the corpus callosum, a constellation of findings termed septo-optic dysplasia, or De Morsier's syndrome. Other less common abnormalities are cortical heterotopia, pachygyria and schizencephaly. Occasional cases

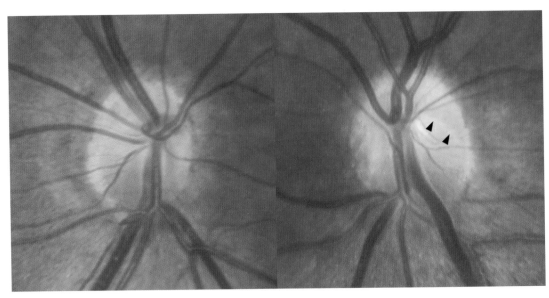

Figure 3.11 Fundus photographs of the above patient with asymptomatic bilateral inferior altitudinal field defects. The upper margin of the true optic disc (arrowheads) is distinct from the edge of the scleral canal. This mismatch is diagnostic of superior segmental hypoplasia.

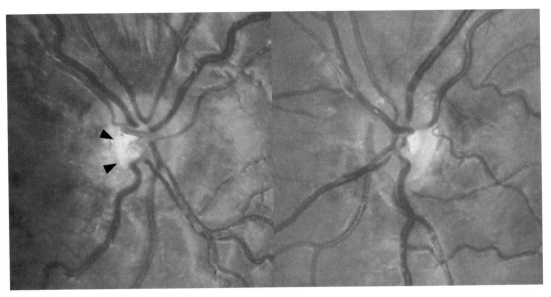

Figure 3.12 Fundus photographs of a child with optic nerve hypoplasia who presented in infancy with poor fixation and nystagmus. The discs are much smaller than the scleral canal (arrowheads indicate true disc margin in the right eye), leaving a variably pigmented gap and creating the classic "double-ring" sign. The right eye is affected more severely than the left.

Table 3.2 Factors associated with an increased risk of optic nerve hypoplasia

Young maternal age
First parity
Smoking
Cytomegalovirus
Toxins
  phenytoin
  lysergic acid diethylamide (LSD)
  phencyclidine (PCP)
  marijuana
  alcohol

of optic nerve hypoplasia are associated with pan-hypopituitarism, even in the absence of other structural brain abnormalities. If unrecognized, such endocrine deficiency can lead to growth retardation, developmental delay, diabetes insipidus and even sudden death. Panhypopituitarism may be predicted by the MRI which, on non-contrast T1-weighted images, typically shows that the normal bright signal of the posterior pituitary gland is either absent or higher than normal, located in the infundibulum.

Unilateral and segmental forms of hypoplasia are generally associated with good visual acuity. Growth delay and endocrine failure are uncommon in these cases. A specific form of partial optic nerve hypoplasia that affects the offspring of insulin-dependent diabetic mothers has been termed *superior segmental hypoplasia* or the *"topless disc syndrome"*. While initially considered to be a rare anomaly, a study of 34 offspring of diabetic mothers found a prevalence of 8.8%. This condition is usually bilateral, affects females more often than males, and is not asso-

ciated with other developmental anomalies. It is rarely present in patients who do not have a history of maternal diabetes. The pathogenesis of superior segmental hypoplasia is unknown and it is particularly puzzling that such a focal deficit should result from a systemic metabolic abnormality. Individuals with this condition are asymptomatic since their visual world has been truncated since birth. Inferior field loss is usually discovered during routine testing, as in our patient, or during the investigation of an unrelated visual problem.

Children with optic nerve hypoplasia should be monitored for signs of developmental delay or growth failure. The risk of these complications is greater in cases with severe bilateral visual loss and in such patients neuro-imaging and endocrinologic evaluation are usually undertaken at the time of diagnosis. In those with partial forms that are discovered in adult life, such as the patient presented here with segmental optic nerve hypoplasia, no ancillary testing is needed.

Diagnosis: Superior segmental hypoplasia

Tip: Superior segmental hypoplasia of the optic disc is a benign congenital anomaly that affects the offspring of diabetic mothers. A critical examination of the fundus is diagnostic.

Incidental abduction deficit

Case: A 45-year-old homemaker had an eye examination because of presbyopic symptoms. In the course of her evaluation it was noted that abduction of the left eye was incomplete (Figure 3.13). She did not experience diplopia but noted that images did

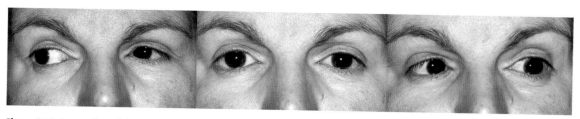

Figure 3.13 Incomplete abduction of the left eye in an asymptomatic 45-year-old homemaker.

look a bit "blurry" when she looked to the left. An MR scan of brain and orbits was unrevealing.

What feature identifies this woman's abduction deficit as a congenital, rather than acquired, sixth nerve palsy?

In addition to incomplete abduction of the left eye there is narrowing of the palpebral fissure and globe retraction when that eye is adducted. This motility pattern indicates a Type I Duane's syndrome, i.e. a form of congenital sixth nerve palsy. The patient was reassured as to the benign nature of this defect.

Discussion: Duane's syndrome is a congenital brainstem anomaly in which there is aberrant innervation of the lateral rectus muscle with resultant co-firing of the ipsilateral medial and lateral rectus muscles. Pathologic studies in this syndrome have shown agenesis of the sixth nerve nucleus with innervation to the lateral rectus muscle supplied instead by branches of the third nerve. This anomalous innervation produces a synkinesis on attempted adduction due to simultaneous activation of the medial and lateral rectus muscles resulting in globe retraction and fissure narrowing. Three subtypes have been defined based on clinical and electromyographic features. *Type I* is the most common form and is characterized by incomplete abduction, as exemplified in this patient. In *Type II,* adduction is impaired, and in *Type III,* both adduction and abduction are incomplete. Duane's syndrome is more common in women and most often affects the left eye, for reasons that are unknown. Other features that may be present in Duane's syndrome include exaggerated elevation or depression of the eye in adduction and A-, V-, or X-pattern ocular deviations. Occasional patients have other forms of anomalous innervation such as a Marcus Gunn jaw-wink or paradoxical-gustatory-lacrimal reflex ("crocodile tears") and some others have developmental anomalies including Goldenhar syndrome, Klippel–Feil anomaly, sensorineural deafness and Wildervanck syndrome (cervico-oculo-acoustic anomaly).

Despite loss of abduction, patients with Type I Duane's syndrome usually remain well aligned in primary position. This clinical feature is extremely helpful for distinguishing this condition from acquired sixth nerve palsy and from other causes of acquired abduction deficit which typically produce esotropia.

Diagnosis: Type I Duane's syndrome

Tip: An abduction deficit that is acquired should produce diplopia. When it does not, a congenital anomaly should be suspected. Look carefully for narrowing of the palpebral fissure and globe retraction when the eye is in adduction.

Intermittent vertical diplopia

Case: A 50-year-old salesman presented with a one-year history of intermittent vertical binocular diplopia unassociated with head or eye pain. His double vision usually occurred at the end of the day when he was tired. He denied other focal neurologic deficits including dysphagia, dysarthria, limb weakness, hoarseness and fatigue with chewing. An MRI of brain and orbits, MRA of the cranial vessels, thyroid function tests, acetylcholine receptor antibodies and results of a lumbar puncture were all normal or negative.

Neuro-ophthalmic examination demonstrated a 10 diopter left hyperphoria in primary position, worse on right gaze and with left head tilt. There was subtle underaction of the left superior oblique with otherwise full extraocular movements. Testing with double Maddox rods indicated five degrees of excyclotorsion OS. Lids and pupils were normal including no fatigability or lid twitch. His examination was consistent with a left superior oblique (fourth nerve) palsy, but investigation for specific causes had been unrevealing. Because of the intermittent nature of his symptoms and worsening of diplopia with fatigue, myasthenia was suspected. A Tensilon (edrophonium chloride) test, however, was negative.

Table 3.3 Causes of fourth nerve palsy

Trauma
Congenital
Idiopathic
Tumor
Brainstem stroke
Demyelinating disease
Increased intracranial pressure
Dural-cavernous fistula
Aneurysm

What other causes of fourth nerve palsy should be considered?

The most common types of fourth nerve palsy are traumatic, congenital and idiopathic (See Table 3.3). At this point, the possibility of a congenital fourth nerve palsy was considered.

How would you pursue a diagnosis of congenital fourth nerve palsy in this patient?

His *vertical fusional amplitudes* were assessed with a prism bar, yielding a measurement of 12 diopters. Such supra-normal fusional capacity is, for practical purposes, diagnostic of a congenital fourth nerve palsy. Inspection of childhood photographs confirmed a pre-existing and long-standing right head tilt. Based on these observations, a diagnosis of congenital right fourth nerve palsy was made. He was treated with spectacle correction that included a total of 6 diopters of prism (3 base up in the right eye, 3 base down in the left) and enjoyed relief of his intermittent diplopia.

Discussion: Common causes of vertical diplopia include cranial nerve palsy (third or fourth), skew deviation, restrictive orbitopathy and myasthenia. Fourth nerve palsy can usually be distinguished from other mechanisms by means of the Bielschowski three-step test, also known as the head tilt test (Figure 3.14). This useful technique is designed to determine the paretic muscle in

patients with vertical diplopia and is performed as follows:

Step 1   Record which is the higher eye in primary position. If the left eye is higher, for example, there is either failure of elevation of the right eye (weakness of the superior rectus or inferior oblique muscle) or failure of depression of the left eye (weakness of the superior oblique or inferior rectus muscle).

Step 2   Note whether the misalignment is greater on left gaze or right gaze. This step is based on the principle that any ocular motor deviation will be worse in the field of action of the paretic muscle. A left hypertropia that is worse on right gaze must be due to weakness of a muscle acting in that field of gaze, thus narrowing down the choices to the right superior rectus or the left superior oblique.

Step 3   Record the direction of head tilt that worsens the deviation. Tilting to the left normally evokes excyclotorsion of the right eye and incyclotorsion of the left eye. Incyclotorsion is normally accomplished by both the superior rectus and superior oblique, whose vertical actions cancel each other. In the presence of superior oblique weakness, however, head tilt toward the involved side evokes the unopposed vertical action of the intact superior rectus, thus further elevating that eye. It is this mechanism that accounts for the third step of the head tilt test. Thus, a patient with left fourth nerve palsy will have a left hyperdeviation in primary position that is worse on right gaze and with left head tilt.

The most common cause of an acquired fourth nerve palsy is trauma (see Table 3.3). The most common non-traumatic mechanism is a congenital anomaly of the superior oblique muscle or its tendon. Congenital fourth nerve palsy often presents in mid-life rather than childhood, not because of worsening muscle weakness, but rather due to progressive loss of fusion. The range of fusional capacity is variable and tends to decline over a lifetime. Individuals with a congenital fourth nerve palsy initially have sufficiently large fusional capacities to

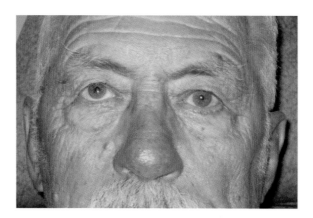

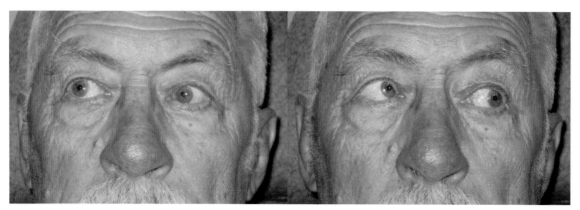

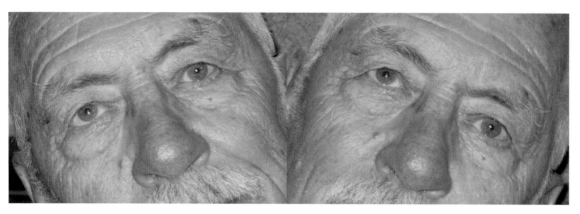

Figure 3.14 The three-step test in a patient with a traumatic right fourth nerve palsy. He has a right hypertropia that is worse on left gaze and with right head tilt.

maintain ocular alignment. Such fusional capacity may diminish as part of the normal aging process, or diminution may be precipitated by exogenous factors such as intercurrent illness, certain central nervous system diseases (particularly Parkinson's disease), pregnancy and the use of drugs that have central nervous system depressant actions such as anti-convulsants, sedative-hypnotics and pain medications. Extensive visual loss also can precipitate breakdown of the fusional mechanism due to loss of sufficient visual field required to maintain binocular fusion. In occasional patients, the onset of diplopia from a decompensated palsy is related to a change in a long-standing compensatory behavior such as the obligatory downgaze imposed by the use of bifocals. We have seen one patient whose congenital fourth nerve palsy became manifest when she was unable to adopt her usual compensatory head tilt following a neck injury.

In all of these instances, when the fusional capacity becomes inadequate, the congenital fourth nerve palsy is said to be decompensated and patients experience diplopia. In most individuals with a decompensated fourth nerve palsy, failure of fusion is initially intermittent, often influenced by fatigue, alcohol and other factors. Because of this apparent variability, patients with a decompensated congenital fourth nerve palsy often are misdiagnosed as myasthenic.

Examination of old photographs (sometimes referred to as Family Album Tomography or a "FAT" scan) can be helpful for establishing the presence of a pre-existing head tilt, which typically accompanies a congenital fourth nerve palsy. Facial asymmetry, with mild relative hypoplasia on the side of the palsy, is also a common finding. In addition, patients with a congenital fourth nerve palsy often have a larger degree of inferior oblique overaction compared to those with acquired palsy. While these findings are supportive evidence for a congenital fourth nerve palsy, the most definitive clinical feature is the demonstration of greater than normal vertical fusional amplitudes. Normal vertical fusional amplitudes range from 2 to 4 diopters but occasionally are a bit larger in patients with a long-standing acquired muscle imbalance. In contrast, patients with a congenital phoria often have huge amplitudes, in some cases easily "marching up" the prism bar to 25 diopters or more. The demonstration of vertical fusional amplitudes greater than 10 diopters is usually considered diagnostic of a congenital palsy and can be enormously helpful for obviating the need for ancillary testing.

Diagnosis: Congenital fourth nerve palsy

Tip: Decompensated congenital fourth nerve palsy often presents as intermittent diplopia that is worse with fatigue, suggesting myasthenia. The demonstration of supra-normal vertical fusional amplitudes is diagnostic of its congenital nature.

FURTHER READING

Pseudopapilledema

A. C. Arnold, Optic disc drusen. *Ophthalmol Clin N Am*, **4** (1991), 505–17.

M. C. Brodsky, Congenital anomalies of the optic disc. In N. R. Miller, N. J. Newman, V. Biousse, J. B. Kerrison, eds., *Walsh and Hoyt's Clinical Neuro-Ophthalmology*, 6th edn. Philadelphia: Lippincott Williams and Wilkins, 2005) Vol. 1, Chapter 3, pp. 151–95.

Superior segmental hypoplasia

R. Y. Kim, W. F. Hoyt, S. Lessell, M. H. Narahara, Superior segmental optic hypoplasia: a sign of maternal diabetes. *Arch Ophthalmol*, **107** (1989), 1312–15.

K. Landau, J. Djahanschahi Bajka, B. M. Kirchschläger, Topless optic disks in children of mothers with type I diabetes mellitus. *Am J Ophthalmol*, **125** (1998), 605–11.

M. Nelson, S. Lessell, A. A. Sadun, Optic nerve hypoplasia and maternal diabetes mellitus. *Arch Neurol*, **43** (1986), 20–5.

Duane's syndrome

P. A. DeRespinis, A. R. Caputo, R. S. Wagner, S. Guo, Duane's retraction syndrome. *Surv Ophthalmol*, **38** (1993), 257–88.

N. R. Miller, S. M. Kiel, W. R. Green, A. W. Clark, Unilateral Duane's retraction syndrome (Type I). *Arch Ophthalmol*, **100** (1982), 1468–72.

Congenital superior oblique palsy

P. W. Brazis, Palsies of the trochlear nerve: diagnosis and localization – recent concepts. *Mayo Clin Proc*, **68** (1993), 501–9.

E. M. Helveston, D. Krach, D. A. Plager, F. D. Ellis, A new classification of superior oblique palsy based on congenital variations in the tendon. *Ophthalmology*, **99** (1992), 1609–15.

G. K. Von Noorden, E. Murray, S. Y. Wong, Superior oblique paralysis. A review of 270 cases. *Arch Ophthalmol*, **104** (1986), 1771–6.

4

Radiographic errors

Neuro-ophthalmology emerged as a subspecialty in the pre-scan era, when a great premium was placed on accurate localization of disease process without resorting to surgical exploration. One aspect of the field that draws many of us to this discipline is just this ability to localize a lesion based solely on the clinical findings. While sometimes viewed as obsolete in today's era of sophisticated neuro-imaging, this skill is particularly valuable for the interpretation of radiographic studies.

In an ideal world, the clinician and the neuroradiologist would read each scan together. In every day life, we often settle for less but at the least, the clinician should always furnish the radiologist with a clear directive regarding the area of interest on the scan and the nature of the suspected disease process. The more confidently the clinician can establish the location of the lesion based on the clinical findings, the more attentive the radiologist can be to the area of interest. And when the scan interpretation is inconsistent with the clinical findings, the scan should be reviewed again.

In this chapter, we have divided some common radiographic errors into three groups and provide several case examples within each category. The first category consists of cases in which the wrong scan has been obtained, i.e. an error on the part of the clinician who ordered the study. In the next two groups, the study was the correct one but the critical radiographic abnormality was missed, i.e. an error by the interpreter of the scan. In the first of these the diagnosis was missed because the key finding was small and subtle. In the other, the finding was not appreciated because it was either bilateral or involved a midline structure, making the interpretation more challenging. In each case, familiarity with the clinical features of the disorder points to the correct diagnosis.

Ordering the wrong scan

The value of any radiographic study is determined in large part by the quality of the scanner, the sophistication of the software and the expertise of the person reading the scan. Even the best quality scan may be inadequate if it is the wrong study for the clinical question at hand.

Progressive optic neuropathy

Case 1: A healthy 57-year-old homemaker described a three-year history of slowly progressive dimming of vision in the left eye. She denied eye pain, diplopia and other focal neurologic deficits. An eye examination early in her course was said to be normal but two years later, a follow-up examination showed left optic disc pallor. An MRI was unrevealing and she received a diagnosis of "chronic optic neuritis".

Is there a problem with the diagnosis of "chronic optic neuritis"?

The answer to this question, and the key to the diagnosis in this case, rests on the time course of the visual loss. What we mean by "chronic" in this

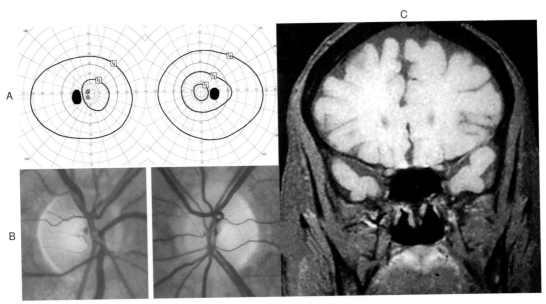

Figure 4.1 Middle-aged woman with progressive dimming of vision in the left eye. (A) The Goldmann visual field is normal in the right eye and shows central depression and two small paracentral scotomas in the left eye. (B) Fundus photographs show a normal right disc and temporal pallor of the left disc. (C) A coronal non-contrast fat-suppressed T1-weighted MR image through the optic canals is normal.

context is not long-standing but showing continued slow progression. Most patients with demyelinating optic neuritis present with acute visual loss, usually progressing over just a few days. Occasional patients with multiple sclerosis develop a subclinical optic neuropathy, and in such cases the patient may not be able to pinpoint an exact onset of visual loss, but the course is not one of continued progression. Less common causes of optic nerve inflammation, such as granulomatous disease, may produce subacute optic neuropathy with progression over weeks to months. In rare cases of optic neuritis due to spirochetal disease, the time course may be more prolonged. In some patients, difficulty in getting a good handle on the temporal features of the visual loss makes the time course indeterminate. For example, we see patients who describe their decreased vision as progressive but actually mean that their visual loss is static but they are worrying about it more. In other cases, a patient with a residual optic neuropathy following a bout of optic neuritis subse-

quently develops another source of decreased acuity such as presbyopia or cataract which makes it appear that optic nerve dysfunction is worsening. Thus, establishing the time course of a patient's optic neuropathy is sometimes challenging. But if the course is well defined and it is one of slowly progressive optic nerve dysfunction, a diagnosis of "chronic optic neuritis" is unlikely to be correct.

Continued progression of this patient's visual loss prompted neuro-ophthalmic referral. Visual acuities were 20/20 OD and 20/70 OS with a moderate (2+) RAPD OS. She identified all 17 color plates in the right eye and just 5 plates in the left eye. Goldmann perimetry in the right eye was normal; in the left eye there was central depression and two small relative scotomas temporal to fixation (Figure 4.1A). The right optic disc was normal, the left showed temporal pallor (Figure 4.1B). Ocular motility was normal and there were no lid abnormalities, proptosis, chemosis or conjunctival injection.

What clinical features in this case suggest the likely mechanism of her chronic optic neuropathy?

In addition to the history of slowly progressive visual loss, the examination furnishes some important clues that point to the correct diagnosis. The earliest and most sensitive signs of optic nerve compression are *decreased color vision* and a *prominent RAPD*. Loss of visual acuity and optic disc pallor are later findings and visual field abnormalities are non-specific. This patient demonstrates the classic clinical features of a compressive optic neuropathy and further work-up should be pursued accordingly.

What additional radiographic evaluation should be obtained?

Her MRI was repeated, this time with contrast, and revealed a small comma-shaped enhancing lesion medial to the left intraorbital optic nerve (Figure 4.2). A diagnosis of optic nerve sheath meningioma was made and the patient received

external beam radiation therapy consisting of 5400 cGy in 30 fractions. Subsequent follow-up visits showed progressive improvement of color vision and pupillary responses, with recovery of acuity to 20/20. Three years after radiation treatment she reported a persistently decreased sense of smell but no other adverse reactions. The patient remains stable clinically and radiographically 12 years later.

Case 2: A 34-year-old administrative assistant experienced a "film" over the vision in her left eye during her 29th week of pregnancy. Two previous pregnancies had been uneventful and she was in otherwise excellent health. Examination showed visual acuities of 20/15 OD and 20/20 OS with mild non-specific depression of visual field in the left eye. Color vision and optic disc appearance were normal but there was a small (1+) RAPD on the left side. An MRI was obtained but without contrast agent because of her pregnancy. There were two small, non-specific lesions in the cerebral white matter; the orbit views were normal. A diagnosis of

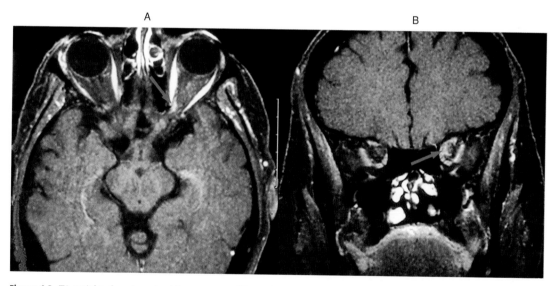

Figure 4.2 T1-weighted post-contrast fat-suppressed MRI of the orbits in the above patient. (A) On the axial image there is a small area of enhancement medial to the optic nerve at the left orbital apex and the anterior aspect of the optic canal (arrow). (B) On a coronal image through the orbital apex this area of abnormal enhancement has a crescentic appearance (arrow). This lesion was not detectable without the use of contrast.

A   B   C

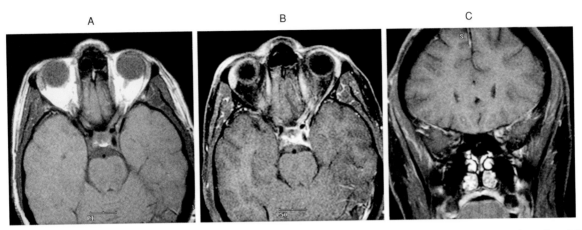

Figure 4.3 MRI of the above patient who developed a left optic neuropathy during pregnancy. (A) Four years later, the axial non-contrast study is still normal. On the T1-weighted post-contrast image with fat suppression there is enhancement (seen on (B) axial and (C) coronal sections) surrounding the posterior left optic nerve (arrow), consistent with an optic nerve sheath meningioma.

idiopathic (demyelinating) optic neuritis was made and she was followed expectantly. Following an uneventful delivery, the vision in her left eye improved spontaneously. Her clinical course was felt to be consistent with the working diagnosis and therefore no additional studies were undertaken.

She remained well until four years later when she experienced recurrent darkening of vision in her left eye. She had been warned of the risk of future multiple sclerosis and she took this recurrent visual loss as a sign of the disease. Based on her belief that nothing could be done, she did not immediately seek medical attention. Her visual loss continued to progress however, and six months later she returned for follow-up. Visual acuity OS was only slightly worse at 20/25 but there was now a large central scotoma and a moderate (2+) left RAPD. An MRI with contrast and fat-suppressed orbit views revealed a small intracanalicular meningioma (Figure 4.3). She received 5400 cGy of external beam radiation in 30 fractions and experienced progressive improvement of vision. Five years later, her vision is stable.

Discussion: Meningiomas are usually isointense to brain on both T1- and T2-weighted images (Figure 4.4). Because of this radiographic charac-

teristic, detection of meningiomas was often difficult prior to the advent of gadolinium. It is important to be aware of this limitation of non-enhanced scans, particularly in the diagnosis of small tumors, whether they are located in the orbit or in the intracranial space. Inclusion of contrast infusion is also important for the detection of orbital inflammation.

In some cases, careful inspection of non-contrast MR images reveals enlargement of the optic nerve silhouette suggesting the presence of a mass lesion, but this is not true in all cases, particularly for intracanalicular lesions. Because there is scant additional room within the optic canal, even a small increase in the size of a tumor in this location can cause relatively rapid and profound loss of vision. In cases of unexplained optic neuropathy, especially those with continued progression, careful scrutiny of this area is crucial. Because the orbital fat normally appears bright on T1- and T2-weighted images, enhancement around the optic nerve is only visible if the study includes dedicated orbital views with fat suppression.

Case 2 also highlights a curious feature of certain compressive lesions: spontaneous regression and resolution. This phenomenon has been previously

A   B

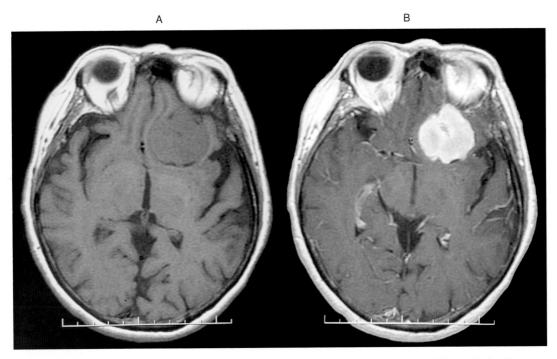

Figure 4.4 Asymptomatic sphenoid wing meningioma found in a middle-aged woman when an MRI was obtained because of a dizzy spell. (A) An axial non-contrast brain MRI shows a round, well circumscribed mass that is isointense to brain on this T1-weighted image. (B) Following contrast administration there is intense, homogeneous enhancement of the tumor.

described in cases of compressive optic neuropathy at the orbital apex and also in patients with sixth nerve palsy. In the case under discussion, tumor regression was likely associated with the vascular and hormonal changes associated with the post-partum state.

Diagnosis: Optic nerve sheath meningioma

Tip: Radiographic evaluation of a progressive, unilateral optic neuropathy is incomplete without a post-contrast fat-suppressed orbital MRI that includes axial and coronal views.

Headache and papilledema

Case: A 25-year-old cashier presented to her local emergency room with a one-week history of severe headache and pulsatile tinnitus. She had been previously healthy and was on no medications. She reported a 10 pound (4.5 kg) weight gain over the preceding year with current weight of 150 pounds (68 kg). Neurologic examination was normal except for bilateral disc edema. Visual acuity, pupillary responses and confrontational visual fields were normal. A CT scan including contrast infusion was unrevealing. Lumbar puncture demonstrated an opening pressure of 360 mm of water in the lateral decubitus position with normal cerebrospinal fluid (CSF) protein, glucose and cell count.

She received a diagnosis of idiopathic intracranial hypertension (IIH) and was started on oral acetazolamide. Neurologic follow-up was scheduled in two weeks, however one week later she returned to the emergency room because of a brief generalized seizure. MRI showed a venous infarct in the left parietal region and a CT venogram demonstrated thrombosis of the left transverse sinus (Figure 4.5).

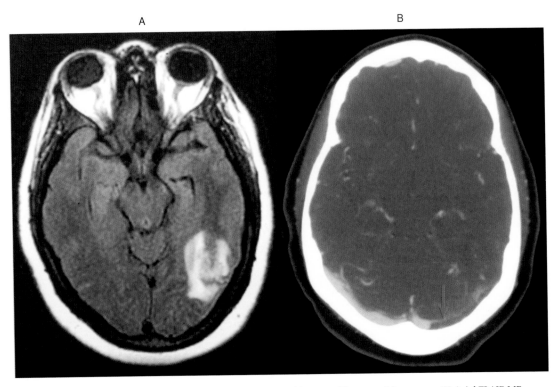

Figure 4.5 Young woman with severe headache, papilledema and increased intracranial pressure. (A) Axial FLAIR MR image shows a left parietal venous infarct. (B) An axial CT venogram shows non-filling of the left transverse sinus (arrow) consistent with thrombosis.

The patient was anticoagulated and subsequently found to have anticardiolipin antibody syndrome.

Discussion: The criteria for the diagnosis of *idiopathic intracranial hypertension* (termed *pseudotumor cerebri* in the older literature) are: elevated intracranial pressure (>250 mm of water in adults and 200 mm in children) with normal CSF constituents, signs and symptoms limited to those of increased intracranial pressure (ICP), and no radiographic evidence of tumor, hydrocephalus or venous sinus occlusion. IIH usually affects otherwise healthy obese women of childbearing age. The mechanism by which obesity produces increased ICP is not completely understood but evidence suggests an abnormality of vitamin A metabolism. Cases fulfilling the diagnostic criteria but due

to a specific identifiable mechanism are sometimes referred to as *secondary* pseudotumor (see Table 4.1). With modern neuro-imaging, the process of ruling out a neoplasm or other mass lesion as the cause of increased ICP is usually straightforward. The identification of cerebral venous sinus thrombosis (CVT) may present more of a challenge.

The severity of clinical signs in patients with CVT depends in large part on the mechanism and the location of the occlusion. Signs and symptoms are usually more fulminant in patients with thrombosis compared to those with mass lesions causing compression of venous structures. Occlusion of the anterior portion of the superior sagittal sinus produces only mild symptoms, whereas involvement of the posterior portion results in severe clinical manifestations. Occlusion of the dominant

Table 4.1 Conditions associated with pseudotumor cerebri syndrome

Endocrine disorders
   obesity
   hypoadrenalism (spontaneous or steroid withdrawal)
   hypoparathyroidism
   growth hormone replacement
   thyroid replacement in children
Toxins
   excessive vitamin A (vitamin, liver, isotretinoin)
   tetracycline, minocycline
   lithium
   chlordecone
   nalidixic acid
Increased cerebral venous pressure
   sinus thrombosis (congenital or acquired
      coagulopathies)
   compression of venous structures
   radical neck dissection
   arteriovenous malformation
Systemic conditions
   uremia
   iron-deficiency anemia
   systemic lupus erythematosus

(usually right) lateral sinus causes markedly increased ICP, whereas occlusion of the non-dominant side may be asymptomatic. Occlusion within the deep venous drainage system (straight sinus or the vein of Galen) usually presents with altered consciousness and long tract signs, and pursues a rapidly downhill course. In contrast, obstruction of the superior sagittal or transverse sinuses may cause signs and symptoms only due to increased ICP. In such cases with normal CSF constituents, the clinical picture may thus mimic IIH.

While CT scanning may reveal abnormalities in patients with CVT, its relative lack of sensitivity limits its usefulness in this condition. On a non-contrast CT, a thrombosed sinus may appear as an abnormally high density within the sinus. This abnormality, however, is identifiable in only 5% of cases. Cerebral edema and areas of hemorrhagic infarction may be seen but are often absent. Follow-ing contrast administration, an "empty delta sign" may be seen, reflecting low-density clot surrounded by a border of enhancement of collateral veins in the sinus wall. While distinctive, this abnormality is found in only about one-third of cases.

In contrast, MR imaging is an extremely sensitive modality for the detection of CVT and has become the technique of choice for the diagnosis and follow-up of such patients. A thrombosed sinus appears hyperintense on T1- and T2-weighted sequences of a routine brain MRI due to accumulation and degradation of hemoglobin. The pitfall of relying on MRI alone is the occurrence of false negative and false positive studies in certain circumstances. A falsely negative MRI, i.e. absence of bright signal in the affected venous structure, can occur if the study is performed very early or very late in the course of sinus thrombosis. In the first two or three days following acute thrombosis, the involved sinus is isointense to brain on T1-weighted images and remains hypointense on T2-weighted images. Later in the course, the sinus may lose its hyperintense signal and regain a more normal appearance, particularly if partial re-canalization has occurred. A false-positive MRI may occur when venous flow is slowed but not thrombosed. In either case, the addition of venography (MR or CT) should help clarify the diagnosis. Post-contrast MR and CT venography (MRV and CTV) are highly sensitive for demonstrating absent or decreased venous flow. These two modalities are comparable in terms of sensitivity.

In the evaluation of patients with increased ICP, CT scanning is usually adequate for excluding a mass lesion and hydrocephalus but is insensitive for the detection of venous sinus thrombosis. CT is also relatively insensitive for the detection of certain other conditions, such as gliomatosis cerebri and meningeal inflammation, that may cause increased ICP without ventriculomegaly or a mass lesion. Consequently post-contrast MRI has generally been considered a requisite for evaluating patients with suspected increased ICP. The addition of MRV or CTV is currently recommended to identify those patients with sinus thrombosis. In one study of patients with presumed IIH who had been imaged only with MRI, the addition of MRV led to the identification of a cerebral venous thrombosis in 10% of cases. Most of these patients, however, did not fit the typical demographic profile of IIH. Such "atypical" patients include men, non-obese women, prepubescent children and patients older than age 44 years.

Diagnosis: Cerebral venous sinus thrombosis

Tip: The investigation of patients with suspected idiopathic intracranial hypertension should include post-contrast MRI. The inclusion of venography is especially important in the evaluation of "atypical" patients.

Idiopathic ptosis and miosis

Case: A 26-year-old law student noticed drooping of his right upper lid for about one year. He had no eye pain, headache or visual symptoms but recently developed brief episodes of tingling in his right cheek, prompting him to seek medical attention. Examination showed 2 mm of right upper lid ptosis without definite lower lid ptosis (Figure 4.6A). There was no lid fatigue or twitch sign. Eye movements were full and saccades were brisk and accurate. In dim room light, pupils measured 4.5 mm OD and 6.0 mm OS. Both pupils constricted briskly to light stimulation but the right pupil exhibited dilation lag in darkness. Pharmacologic testing with 1% apraclonidine showed retraction of the upper lid and pupillary dilation on the right side, consistent with adrenergic denervation supersensitivity (Figure 4.6B). He returned one week later for hydroxyamphetamine testing. After instillation of two drops of 1% hydroxyamphetamine in each eye, there was dilation of the left pupil but no response in the right pupil (Figure 4.6C).

A diagnosis of postganglionic Horner syndrome was made. An MRI of the brain with views of the craniocervical junction was normal (Figure 4.7). The patient was satisfied with a diagnosis of idiopathic Horner syndrome, especially as it had been a year since onset and he continued to feel well in other respects. However his grandfather, who was

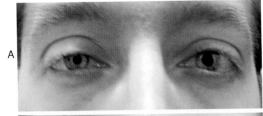
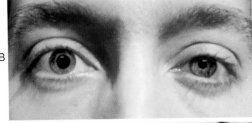
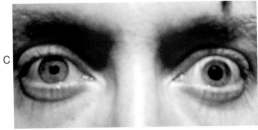

Figure 4.6 Young man with a right Horner syndrome. (A) Baseline examination in dim illumination shows mild right upper lid ptosis and a smaller pupil on the right side. (B) In room light, following instillation of topical apraclonidine in each eye, there is dilation of the right pupil and retraction of the right lid, consistent with adrenergic denervation supersensitivity. There is no appreciable effect of apraclonidine in the left eye. Note that the anisocoria now appears "reversed". (C) Following instillation of topical hydroxyamphetamine in each eye (at a separate visit), there is pupillary dilation and lid retraction on the left side but no response on the right. The asymmetric response to hydroxyamphetamine localizes the patient's right Horner syndrome to the postganglionic sympathetic fibers.

a retired radiologist, requested neuro-ophthalmic consultation.

Why is the current study incomplete?

The sympathetic pathway to the eye is an ipsilateral, three-neuron pathway (Figure 4.8). The

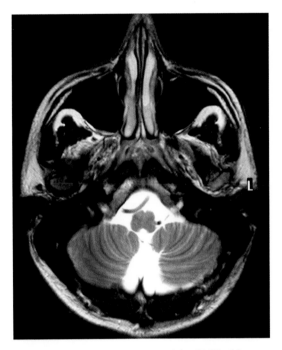

Figure 4.7 Axial non-contrast T2-weighted MRI of the above patient with a right postganglionic Horner syndrome of undetermined etiology. There is no abnormality of the carotid artery or brainstem. The remainder of the scan was also normal.

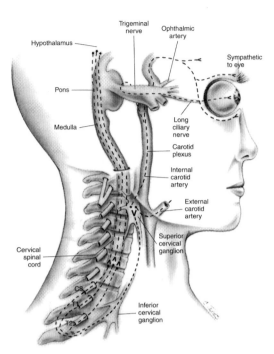

Figure 4.8 Schematic diagram of the sympathetic innervation to the pupil and eyelids. (From G. T. Liu, N. J. Volpe, S. L. Galetta. *Neuro-Ophthalmology, Diagnosis and Management* (Philadelphia: W. B. Saunders, 2001), page 430, with permission.)

first-order (central) neuron descends from the hypothalamus to synapse in the intermediolateral gray column of the cervicothoracic spinal cord. The *second-order (preganglionic) neuron* exits with the ventral rootlets of C8–T2, passes across the apex of the lung and ascends in the neck via the sympathetic chain to synapse in the superior cervical ganglion. The *third-order (postganglionic) neuron* that supplies the pupillodilator and tarsal muscles travels with the internal carotid artery as a plexus around its wall and re-enters the intracranial space via the carotid canal and foramen lacerum. In the cavernous sinus, the oculosympathetic fibers briefly join with the abducens nerve and, once through the orbital apex, follow the nasociliary nerve to the eye.

This patient has a painless, postganglionic Horner syndrome and an unrevealing brain MRI. Keeping

in mind the pathway of the sympathetic fibers to the eye, it should be clear that a complete radiographic investigation should include views down to the level of the superior cervical ganglion. A second MRI with *neck* images was obtained and revealed a large hypervascular lesion at the bifurcation of the right carotid artery (Figure 4.9). The patient underwent an excisional biopsy, which revealed the lesion to be a paraganglioma.

Discussion: Horner syndrome is caused by interruption of the sympathetic innervation to the head and eye producing miosis, ptosis and facial anhidrosis on the side of the lesion. Upper and lower lid ptosis results from superior and inferior tarsal muscle weakness. However, drooping of the lid is generally mild and about 12% of patients with

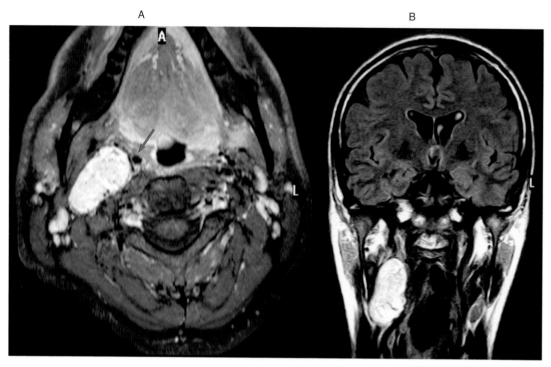

Figure 4.9 Post-contrast fat-suppressed T1-weighted axial image (A) and coronal non-contrast FLAIR image (B) of the neck in the above patient with a right postganglionic Horner syndrome. There is an intensely enhancing lobular lesion in the right neck displacing the carotid artery medially (arrow).

Horner syndrome do not have clinically apparent ptosis. Facial anhidrosis is seldom reported by patients. Thus, anisocoria is the most consistent sign of an oculosympathetic defect. The feature that best defines the anisocoria as oculosympathetic deficiency is *dilation lag* of the smaller pupil in darkness. When the room light is abruptly turned off, the Horner pupil shows slow and delayed dilation over 15–20 seconds compared to the normal pupil which promptly re-dilates back to baseline within 5 seconds. When dilation lag is absent, confirmation of Horner syndrome is provided by pharmacologic testing. The two most commonly used agents for this purpose are cocaine and apraclonidine (see Table 4.2).

Etiologies of Horner syndrome are varied, and their frequency depends on the location of the oculosympathetic defect. Central Horner syndrome is usually due to stroke (e.g. Wallenberg lateral medullary syndrome) and is accompanied by other symptoms and signs of brainstem dysfunction. Preganglionic Horner syndrome is often due to a neoplasm of the pulmonary apex, mediastinum or neck, identified in 20–50% of cases. Postganglionic oculosympathetic defects are commonly accompanied by ipsilateral head/face pain. The most common causes are carotid artery dissection, skull base tumors, lesions in the cavernous sinus and cluster headache.

Any patient with an unexplained Horner syndrome should undergo neuro-imaging to rule out a structural lesion. Localization of the lesion using the hydroxyamphetamine test helps to direct the imaging studies appropriately. If both pupils dilate to hydroxyamphetamine, the Horner syndrome is central or preganglionic; if the Horner pupil does not

Table 4.2 Pharmacologic testing for the diagnosis of Horner syndrome

Agent	Mechanism of Action	Test Procedure	Effect on Normal Eye	Effect on Denervated Eye	Positive Result
Cocaine (4% or 10%)	Inhibition of reuptake of norepinephrine at postsynaptic junction	Put 2 drops in both eyes. Wait 45 minutes	Pupil dilation, lid retraction, conjunctival blanching	None	Anisocoria of 1.0 mm or more (smaller pupil is Horner pupil)
Apracloni-dine (0.5% or 1%)	Weak agonist of post-synaptic alpha 1 adrenergic receptors	Put 1 drop in both eyes. Wait 45 minutes	None	Pupil dilation, lid retraction, conjunctival blanching	Reversal of anisocoria (larger pupil is Horner pupil)

dilate as well as the normal pupil then the lesion is a postganglionic one. Attention to other localizing signs and symptoms is important. If brainstem signs are present, an MRI of the brain with contrast is sufficient. If brainstem signs are absent, then a study of the head, neck and chest should be obtained. Preganglionic Horner syndrome due to apical lung tumor is typically accompanied by ipsilateral arm pain due to infiltration of the brachial plexus. Postganglionic Horner syndrome commonly presents as an isolated finding, usually accompanied by ipsilateral head/face pain. In such cases the evaluation should include MR images of the *head and neck* and MRA with particular attention to the internal carotid artery.

A similar pitfall may occur in the evaluation of increased ICP. Most cases of increased ICP are due to a disease process within the cranial cavity and if the causative lesion is structural an appropriate scan of the head will reveal it. An important exception to this is the patient with a compressive mass in the neck producing obstruction of the venous outflow from the head (Figure 4.10). In such cases the diagnosis may be missed if radiographic studies do not include views of the neck as well as the head.

Diagnosis: Postganglionic Horner syndrome

Tip: Investigation of a postganglionic Horner syndrome should include MR imaging of head and neck in order to visualize the area of the superior cervical ganglion and carotid bifurcation.

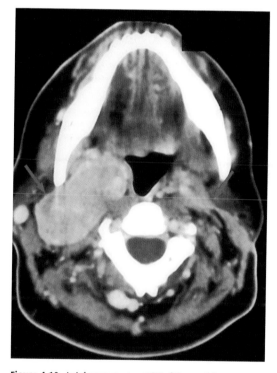

Figure 4.10 Axial post-contrast CT of the neck in a different patient with increased intracranial pressure. There are bilateral paragangliomas, right greater than left (arrows), compressing the right jugular vein and producing a secondary pseudotumor syndrome. This is another example of a case in which the diagnosis would be missed if imaging were restricted to the head.

Subtle radiographic findings

Some radiographic abnormalities are difficult to detect because they are small or subtle. In such cases it is particularly important for the clinician to have a strong suspicion regarding the location and nature of the lesion and to communicate this effectively to the neuroradiologist. In these cases the "trick" to reading the scan is knowing what *should* be there.

"Boxer" ptosis

Case: A 45-year-old factory worker was "headbutted" by her boxer dog while bending over, striking her on the right cheek and throwing her upward and back. The next day she developed a "black eye" with some local tenderness. The discoloration faded over the next week, but just as it was almost gone she developed moderately severe pain behind the right eye that extended to the temple and vertex. Two days later, right upper lid ptosis was noticed by a co-worker.

Examination showed normal afferent visual function and ocular motility. The right pupil measured 3 mm in dim illumination and 2 mm in bright light, the left 5 mm in dim and 2.5 mm in bright light. Both pupils reacted briskly to light but the right pupil showed a delayed response to dark (dilation lag). There was 2 mm of right upper lid ptosis and mild "reverse" lower lid ptosis (Figure 4.11A). Instillation of hydroxyamphetamine produced 3 mm of pupillary dilation on the left side only. An MR scan of head, neck and orbits was reportedly normal.

The above clinical findings are characteristic of a postganglionic Horner syndrome. How might this be related to her preceding trauma?

When the patient was struck by her dog she was thrown back, causing brief but forceful hyperextension of her neck. This form of neck trauma can produce a shearing injury to the internal carotid artery with subsequent dissection, thus causing damage

to the oculosympathetic fibers. Careful examination of her MRI revealed a hyperintense crescent adjacent to the left internal carotid artery on the axial T2-weighted image, characteristic of dissection (Figure 4.11B). An MRA showed some irregularity of the cervical arteries consistent with fibromuscular dysplasia (Figure 4.11C). This underlying vasculopathy presumably rendered her arteries susceptible to damage from relatively trivial trauma.

Discussion: Most cases of acute, painful, postganglionic Horner syndrome are due to carotid dissection or cluster headache. The non-remitting nature of the pain in dissection should help to distinguish these patients from those with cluster headache. Patients with cluster headache typically experience abrupt episodes of pain, frequently occurring during the night and lasting 45–60 minutes. These painful attacks are often associated with a Horner syndrome, which is usually transient but may become permanent after repeated episodes. In some affected individuals, cluster attacks are precipitated by ingestion of alcohol and, for reasons that remain obscure, sufferers often prefer to pace about during their attacks rather than resting in bed.

In contrast, the pain of internal carotid artery (ICA) dissection is unremitting. Pain, which may be localized to the head, eye, jaw, face or neck, is present in over 90% of patients and may be the only manifestation. Scalp tenderness may occur, suggesting a diagnosis of giant cell arteritis (GCA). A postganglionic Horner syndrome occurs in up to 58% of patients with carotid dissection and can be the presenting manifestation.

Transient monocular blindness is reported by about 30% of patients with ICA dissection and is probably caused by decreased perfusion secondary to reduction of the carotid lumen rather than by retinal emboli. Episodes of transient monocular visual loss due to dissection are often precipitated by postural change and may be associated with positive visual phenomena including sparkles and scintillations. ICA dissection can produce retinal emboli but this is rare, probably because of

A

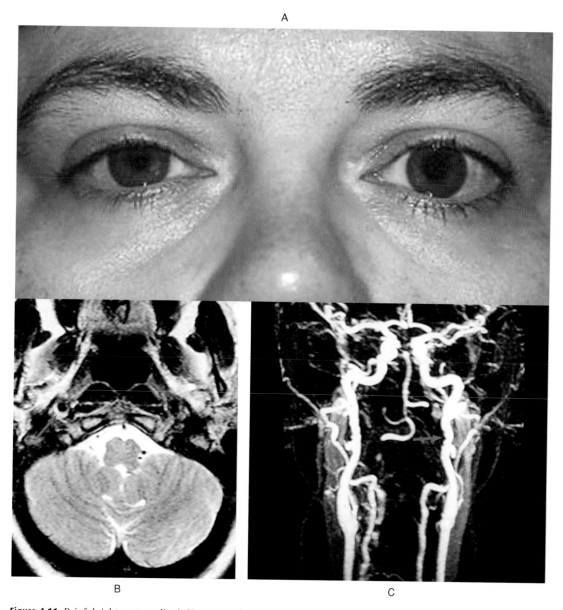

B   C

Figure 4.11 Painful right postganglionic Horner syndrome. (A) External photograph shows miosis and mild upper and lower lid ptosis on the right. (B) Axial T2-weighted MRI shows a hyperintense crescent around the right internal carotid artery (arrow). (C) MRA of cervical and intracranial vessels shows several areas of irregularity consistent with fibromuscular dysplasia (arrow).

reversal of flow through the ophthalmic artery, and permanent visual loss is distinctly uncommon. On the other hand, the incidence of stroke associated with carotid dissection is high, ranging from 12 to 40%. The risk of stroke is highest in the initial two weeks following dissection and diminishes considerably thereafter. If a patient is seen during this time, anticoagulation should be considered, initially with heparin and then with warfarin. Patients who are evaluated one month or more after the acute event can usually be treated with anti-platelet agents alone.

Traumatic dissections are usually due to severe blunt head or neck injury such as motor vehicle accidents, fistfights, hanging, surgery or manipulative neck therapy. Many cases of so-called "spontaneous" dissection may actually have a traumatic origin as well, though the precipitating event may seem trivial, such as coughing, sneezing, childbirth, athletic activities, painting a ceiling, carrying a heavy load or riding a roller coaster. Some patients with spontaneous dissection have an identifiable predisposing disorder such as fibromuscular dysplasia, Marfan's syndrome, Ehlers–Danlos syndrome, alpha-1 antitrypsin deficiency, cystic medical necrosis, syphilis or vasculitis.

Most cases of dissection can be diagnosed with non-invasive methods, including MRI, MR angiography (MRA), CT angiography (CTA) and carotid Dopplers. The study of choice is an axial T1- or T2-weighted pre-contrast MRI of the head that includes images down to the carotid bifurcation. On such images, dissection appears as a bright crescent-shaped signal around the ICA due to the hyperintense signal of methemoglobin within the vessel wall. Significant narrowing of the lumen, when present, is better documented with MRA or by conventional angiography, and appears as the "string sign". Because angiographic methods (whether by catheter study, MRA or CTA) visualize blood flow, dissections that do not impinge on the lumen may not be demonstrable with these techniques but are better identified with MR images, as illustrated by the above case.

Diagnosis: Internal carotid artery dissection

Tip: An acute, postganglionic Horner syndrome with persistent pain is usually due to internal carotid artery dissection. Careful inspection of axial T1- or T2-weighted MR images will reveal the characteristic bright crescent around the artery.

Headache and bilateral third nerve palsy

Case: This 38-year-old, previously healthy maintenance man presented to the emergency room because of chest pain, for which he received tissue thromboplastin activator. The following day he experienced severe headache, photophobia and diplopia. Neurologic examination showed bilateral third nerve palsies, more severe on the right side, and a CT scan was read as normal (Figure 4.12).

What is the diagnosis? What confirmative study would you order?

The abrupt onset of headache and bilateral third nerve palsy is strongly suggestive of pituitary apoplexy, particularly following the use of a thrombolytic agent. This patient's facial features (prominent chin and brow) are characteristic of acromegaly and suggest the presence of a long-standing pituitary tumor. An MRI was obtained, confirming a suprasellar mass with cavernous sinus invasion and hemorrhage (Figure 4.13). In retrospect, his previous CT scan also showed soft tissue in the suprasellar cistern that had been overlooked. Endocrine evaluation showed pituitary insufficiency and elevated growth hormone levels. He was treated with steroids and underwent transphenoidal subtotal resection of his pituitary tumor. Follow-up three months later showed partial recovery of third nerve function.

Discussion: Hemorrhage or infarction of the pituitary gland, usually due to an underlying tumor, is termed *pituitary apoplexy*. This condition typically affects adults and has a wide range of clinical

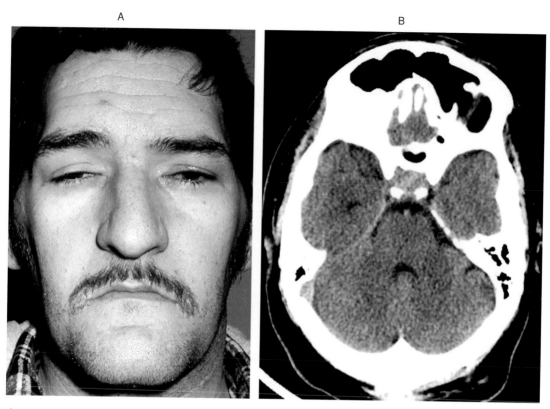

Figure 4.12 (A) A 38-year-old man with abrupt onset of headache and bilateral third nerve palsies. (B) Axial pre-contrast CT of the head read as normal (CT courtesy of Dr. Bradley Robottom).

presentations. Most patients experience abrupt onset of severe headache with symptoms and signs related to meningeal irritation. Some patients also exhibit altered mental status, cranial neuropathy and visual loss due to chiasmal compression. The presence of nuchal rigidity, photophobia and reduced level of consciousness in some patients with this condition may be mistakenly attributed to an aneurysmal subarachnoid hemorrhage or infectious meningitis. Visual loss may be unilateral or bilateral with variable severity. Clouding of consciousness may preclude detailed visual testing; when such testing is possible, a bitemporal pattern of loss is characteristic. Ophthalmoplegia, due to compression of the ocular motor nerves in the cavernous sinus, is also common and may also be uni-

lateral or bilateral. The third nerve is most commonly affected, followed by the sixth and fourth cranial nerves. The advent of high-resolution MR scanning now allows the detection of hemorrhage into a pituitary tumor in occasional patients who have minimal or no symptoms. Strictly speaking, such patients can be classified as having pituitary apoplexy although some authors reserve the term apoplexy for those with a dramatic clinical presentation as described above.

In the majority of cases of apoplexy, the presence of a pituitary tumor was unsuspected prior to hemorrhage. In approximately one-third of patients some sort of precipitating factor is identified. These precipitating events are quite varied, including reduced blood flow to the pituitary gland (as

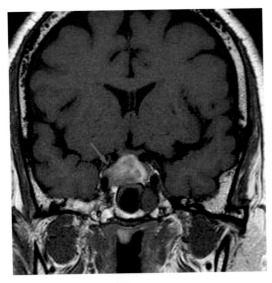

Figure 4.13 MRI of the above patient. Coronal non-contrast T1-weighted image reveals a sellar mass extending into the suprasellar cistern, just contacting but not compressing the optic chiasm. Heterogeneous signal intensity within the mass is consistent with hemorrhage from pituitary apoplexy. The mass extends into the cavernous sinuses, more pronounced on the right side (arrow) (courtesy of Dr. Bradley Robottom).

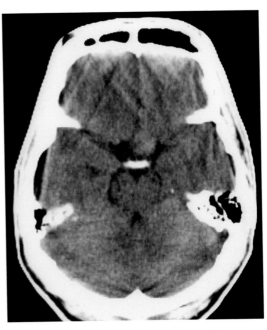

Figure 4.14 CT scan of another patient with pituitary apoplexy causing severe headache, acute bilateral visual loss and ophthalmoplegia. Note the distortion of the suprasellar cistern anteriorly, which is due to filling of this CSF space by infarcted pituitary tissue (arrow).

from hypotension or Valsalva maneuver), an acute increase in blood flow (as in malignant hypertension), stimulation of the pituitary gland (such as pregnancy or with exogenous estrogen administration), emboli from carotid artery surgery, and coagulopathy (from thrombocytopenia, administration of anticoagulant drugs, and thrombolytic agents as in the case under discussion). The occurrence of sudden headache and visual symptoms (afferent and/or efferent) in any of these settings should suggest the possibility of pituitary apoplexy. Because of its varied clinical presentations and at times ambiguous or subtle radiographic findings, a delayed diagnosis of pituitary apoplexy is not uncommon.

Although a standard head CT is usually the most easily accessed radiographic study in an emergency room setting, this imaging study is less effective than MRI for the detection of pituitary apoplexy. CT is often degraded at bone to soft tissue interfaces and is thus less sensitive for visualizing lesions at the skull base. In addition, the suprasellar cistern is a midline structure and therefore detection of an abnormality depends on the examiner's familiarity with its normal appearance. On CT the suprasellar cistern appears as a low density five-sided hypodense area anterior to the midbrain. In many cases the presence of a tumor is manifest not as a visible mass, but as filling in of this CSF-filled space (Figure 4.14). MRI, in contrast, is much better suited for the detection of tumors in this region, and is thus the study of choice in cases of suspected pituitary apoplexy.

Prompt diagnosis of pituitary apoplexy is crucial because these patients are at risk for the systemic complications of acute adrenal insufficiency. Acute management should include the administration of systemic corticosteroids in stress dosages (e.g.

hydrocortisone 100 mg intravenously every six to eight hours) with careful monitoring of electrolyte balance. Surgical decompression is usually indicated although occasional patients do well with conservative management.

Diagnosis: Pituitary apoplexy

Tip: CT is not adequate for ruling out suspected pituitary apoplexy.

Progressive sixth nerve palsy

Case: A 66-year-old retired businessman initially noticed "fuzzy vision" whenever he looked to the left. Over the next month this fuzzy image split into two distinct images. At first he was able to fuse the two images with effort but over the next three months, this became increasingly difficult and he developed consistent diplopia on left gaze. Eventually he experienced diplopia in primary position as well, initially at distance and then at near. He reported no head or eye pain but described a "tired feeling" in his left eye after prolonged distance viewing, such as driving. His past medical history was positive only for benign prostatic hypertrophy. Afferent visual function, pupillary examination and fundus appearance were normal in each eye. He had a 12 diopter esotropia in primary position that increased on left gaze. There was mild limitation of abduction of the left eye and slowing of left lateral rectus saccades, even with small amplitude movements. An MR scan of brain and orbits was reportedly normal (Figure 4.15).

What aspect of this patient's presentation provides the most compelling diagnostic clue?

This patient provides a clear history of gradually progressive diplopia and his examination points to a unilateral cranial nerve palsy. This combination of clinical findings strongly indicates a compressive lesion as the cause. Careful inspection of his MRI focusing on the course of the left sixth nerve revealed a very small enhancing mass at the

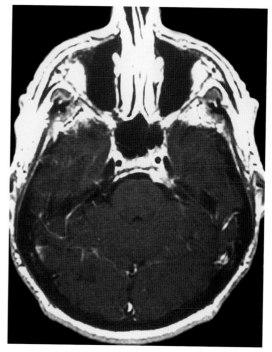

Figure 4.15 Axial post-contrast T1-weighted MR image of a retired businessman with a progressive left sixth nerve palsy, interpreted as normal.

entrance to Dorello's canal, a bony space at the tip of the temporal bone which encloses the abducens nerve as it enters the cavernous sinus (Figure 4.16). A second, small extra-axial focus of enhancement was identified along the upper lateral left cerebral convexity. The radiographic appearance of these lesions was sufficiently characteristic that a diagnosis of meningioma was made without histopathologic confirmation. He was managed initially with prism correction but over the next six months his esotropia increased to 25 diopters. He was then treated with external beam radiation consisting of 5580 cGy in twice-daily fractions. His esotropia subsequently stabilized and he eventually underwent extraocular surgery with good post-operative ocular alignment.

Discussion: In a certain sense, diplopia is always sudden in onset regardless of mechanism; the

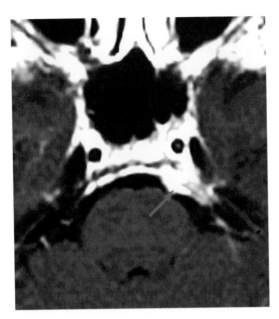

Figure 4.16 Close-up view of the scan shown in Figure 4.15 shows a small enhancing mass at the entrance to Dorello's canal on the left (arrow), consistent with a meningioma.

eyes are either aligned or they are not. Occasional patients, however, describe a definite history of gradual progression, as in the case under discussion. When due to a sixth nerve palsy, such progressive diplopia is initially present only on extreme lateral gaze, eventually progressing to involve center gaze, first at distance and then increasingly at near. Very small angle misalignments are often experienced as blurring rather than doubling of images. When just at the threshold of fusion, diplopia is often intermittent, then, when fusional capacity is exceeded, diplopia becomes constant. For many people, the most frequent visual task that they perform at distance is driving, and so patients with early or mild sixth nerve weakness often experience intermittent horizontal diplopia only during this activity.

The most common mechanism of a sixth nerve palsy in this patient's age group is ischemia, either due to a vasculopathic cranial mononeuropathy or a brainstem stroke. The significance of his history of slow progression is that it rules out an ischemic mechanism. The story in this case so strongly suggests a compressive lesion that a critical view of the scan with attention to the course of the sixth nerve is mandatory. The usual method for doing this is to start at the brainstem and work out to the orbit, tracing the pathway of the involved nerve. The abducens nerve exits the brainstem at the pontomedullary junction and ascends the subarachnoid space along the clivus. It then passes near the inferior petrosal sinus and slides under the petrosphenoid ligament, entering Dorello's canal where it is tethered to the dura. The nerve proceeds through the cavernous sinus to the superior orbital fissure, entering the orbit to innervate the lateral rectus muscle. Axial T1-weighted images without and with contrast are most useful for evaluating the course of the cisternal and petrous portions of the abducens nerve, whereas coronal images provide critical information in the parasellar and orbital segments. Using this technique in the above case, and armed with the conviction (based on the history) that a mass lesion was present, the responsible lesion was identified.

Diagnosis: Petrous ridge meningioma

Tip: Any patient with a slowly progressive sixth nerve palsy should be assumed to harbor a mass lesion.

Midline and bilateral abnormalities

Radiographic abnormalities are most easily identified when the changes are unilateral or asymmetric. Disorders that involve midline structures and those that are bilateral and symmetric may escape detection. The next three cases illustrate this principle.

Bilateral idiopathic sixth nerve palsy

Case: A 62-year-old school psychologist experienced abrupt onset of horizontal diplopia on left gaze. She had no head or eye pain and no other neurologic deficits or recent systemic symptoms.

She took medications for hypertension and hyper-cholesterolemia and was otherwise in good health. Examination one week after onset showed an isolated left abduction deficit. An MR scan was reportedly normal and a presumptive diagnosis of vasculopathic (ischemic) sixth nerve palsy was made (see Chapter 11, Acute isolated sixth nerve palsy). On re-examination one week later she had developed an abduction deficit on the right side as well. There were no other neurologic deficits and no papilledema. An edrophonium chloride (Tensilon) test was said to be equivocal. A lumbar puncture showed an opening pressure of 160 mm of water with normal chemistries, cell count, cytology and flow cytometry. A number of blood tests for vasculitis and systemic inflammatory disease, a chest X-ray and urinalysis were all normal.

Is a diagnosis of vasculopathic sixth nerve palsy still tenable here?

While vasculopathic cranial neuropathy is the most common cause of sixth nerve deficit in individuals over age 50 years, such palsies are virtually always unilateral. A diagnosis of bilateral vasculopathic or idiopathic sixth nerve palsy indicates that the actual cause has not yet been identified.

In light of her negative work-up, the patient was referred for neuro-ophthalmic consultation. Examination showed normal afferent visual function and optic disc appearance. There was a 40 diopter esotropia in primary position with no abduction of either eye past midline and with marked slowing of lateral rectus saccades bilaterally. A second Tensilon test was unequivocally negative.

What are the most common causes of bilateral sixth nerve palsy and what mechanism is most likely in this case?

Processes that frequently affect both sixth nerves include structural lesions at the skull base, disorders of intracranial pressure (too high or too low) and meningitis (See Table 4.3). The two abducens nerves travel in close proximity in the subarach-

Table 4.3 Causes of bilateral sixth nerve palsy

Trauma
Meningitis
Increased intracranial pressure
Low pressure syndromes (post-lumbar puncture, myelography)
Skull base tumor
Pituitary apoplexy
Giant cell arteritis
Wernicke's encephalopathy
Miller Fisher syndrome

noid space, where they are vulnerable to meningeal infiltration (inflammatory or neoplastic), and along the clivus, where they are prone to compression by tumorous expansion. The sixth nerves are particularly vulnerable to changes in intracranial pressure because they are tethered at their entrance into Dorello's canal, so that shifts in brain position due to pressure cause traction. The appropriate work-up for bilateral sixth nerve palsy emerges from these anatomic considerations, and should include high quality neuro-imaging with attention to the skull base, and lumbar puncture, with measurement of intracranial pressure as well as cytologic CSF examination.

Re-evaluation of this patient's MRI disclosed mild expansion of the clivus (Figure 4.17). A transphenoidal biopsy of the lesion revealed a large B-cell lymphoma. A metastatic survey showed no evidence of malignancy elsewhere and she was treated with chemotherapy and external beam radiation. Over the next six months, abduction improved in each eye, but she still had a 16 diopter esotropia in primary position for which she underwent extraocular muscle surgery. Post-operative ocular alignment was excellent and she remained clinically and radiographically stable three years later.

Discussion: Radiographic investigation of the skull base can be challenging. Standard CT sequences have poor resolution in this region due to signal degradation at soft tissue to bone interfaces. MR images are not hampered by this limitation but do

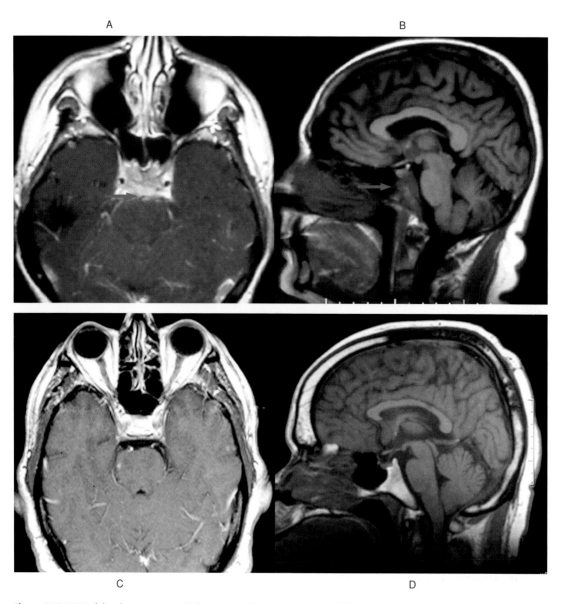

Figure 4.17 MRI of the above patient with bilateral sixth nerve palsy. (A) Axial post-contrast T1-weighted image shows symmetric expansion of the clivus causing loss of the normal pre-pontine cistern (arrow). (B) Sagittal non-contrast image demonstrates expansion of the clivus with an abnormally low signal (dark appearance) (arrow). (C) and (D) are comparable images of a normal subject for purposes of comparison. Notice the sharply defined margins and bright signal of the normal clivus on the sagittal view.

A   B

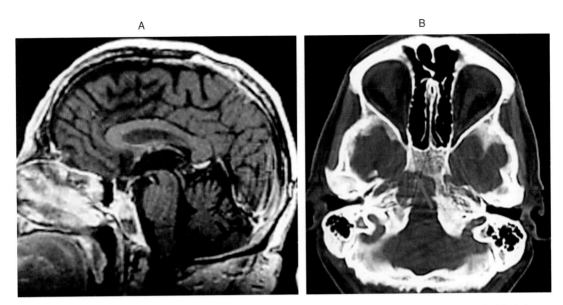

Figure 4.18 Additional examples of skull base metastases involving the clivus in two patients who presented with sixth nerve palsy. (A) Post-contrast T1-weighted sagittal MR image of a patient with multiple myeloma shows loss of the normal bright signal inferiorly within the clivus as well as marked enhancement of its superior aspect. (B) Axial CT of the skull base with bone windows in a patient with renal cell carcinoma reveals a lytic lesion within the right side of the clivus and petrous apex (arrow). The tumor itself is not visible but its presence is inferred because of the missing bone.

not visualize calcium, and so some bony abnormalities may be missed. If a skull base tumor is suspected, adequate radiographic investigation may require both an MRI and a CT with bone windows to fully define the site of origin of the tumor and its soft tissue extension.

Lesions of the clivus can be particularly difficult to appreciate because it is a midline structure and thus comparison of the affected with the normal side is not an option. The normal adult clivus contains red marrow and fatty marrow in varying proportions. On a pre-contrast T1-weighted image, red marrow appears as low-signal intensity (dark) and fatty marrow as high-signal intensity (bright) (Figure 4.17D). In young adults, the clivus has a predominantly low signal with spotty amounts of bright signal; with advancing age, the amount of low signal intensity decreases. In most adults over age 50, the clivus has a predominantly bright signal due to a preponderance of yellow marrow. When invaded by tumor, the clivus instead has a low-signal intensity, and fol-

lowing contrast administration the tumor portion enhances intensely. Normal clival tissue enhances mildly, if at all. In most cases, the clivus is best assessed on mid-sagittal cuts.

Lesions that develop in the clivus include chordoma, chondrosarcoma, plasmacytoma, giant cell tumors, hemangiomas, lymphomas, adenocystic and nasopharyngeal carcinomas and Paget's disease. The clivus is also a site for bony metastases (Figure 4.18). In an older man with prostate cancer, a painless, progressive sixth nerve palsy must be considered a clival metastasis until proven otherwise. In addition to unilateral or bilateral sixth nerve palsy, lesions of the clivus can cause bulbar symptoms due to cranial nerve palsy, brainstem compression and endocrinopathies due to pituitary insufficiency.

Diagnosis: Clivus tumor

Tip: Investigation of unexplained bilateral sixth nerve palsy should include a critical evaluation of the clivus, best assessed on mid-sagittal MRI sections.

Atypical pseudotumor cerebri syndrome

Case: A 62-year-old, previously healthy, non-obese homemaker developed acute onset of severe headache with diplopia and transient obscurations of vision. Examination showed marked bilateral papilledema and mild left sixth nerve paresis (Figure 4.19). An MRI was said to be normal and a lumbar puncture in the lateral decubitus position revealed an opening pressure of 360 mm of water with normal protein, glucose and cell count. A diagnosis of idiopathic intracranial hypertension (IIH) was made and she was started on acetazolamide.

What features of this case are atypical for a diagnosis of IIH? What alternative diagnosis should be considered?

This patient is postmenopausal and not overweight, whereas IIH typically affects obese women of childbearing age. The diagnosis of IIH in a patient who does *not* fit this demographic profile should prompt additional investigation for an identifiable cause of increased intracranial pressure before labeling it as idiopathic (Table 4.4). In particular, cerebral venous sinus occlusion should be the first consideration,

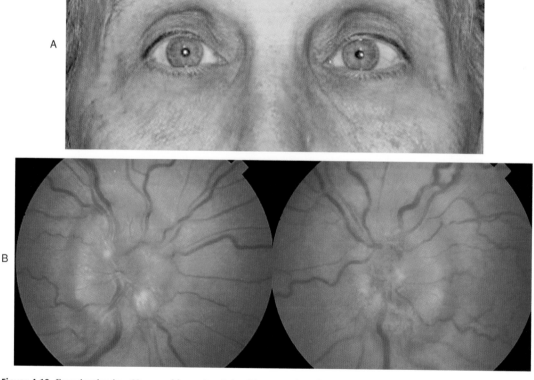

Figure 4.19 Examination in a 62-year-old, previously healthy, non-obese homemaker with acute headache and diplopia shows mild (A) esotropia and (B) bilateral papilledema.

Table 4.4 Laboratory evaluation in patients with cerebral venous sinus thrombosis

Inherited thrombophilias
  anti-thrombin III
  protein S and C
  activated protein C resistance (factor V Leiden mutation)
  prothrombin gene mutation
  homocysteine
  hemoglobin electrophoresis
Acquired pro-thrombotic states
  CBC with platelets
  PT/PTT
  fibrinogen
  serum protein electrophoresis
  antiphospholipid antibodies
  renal function tests
  urinalysis
  cryoglobulins
  search for occult malignancy

and the radiographic studies examined critically with this in mind.

In this case, review of the patient's MRI in fact revealed bright signal in the superior sagittal sinus on both coronal and axial views, indicating sub-acute clot (Figure 4.20). Laboratory investigation disclosed a platelet count of 750 000, leading to a diagnosis of essential thrombocytosis. (See Chapter 5, Empty sella, for further discussion of radiographic findings in IIH.)

Discussion: The clinical features of cerebral venous sinus thrombosis (CVT) depend on several factors, including the site and extent of thrombosis, the rapidity of its evolution and the age of the patient. The most common presentation of CVT consists of new onset of headache with a focal neurologic deficit or a partial seizure. In up to one-third of cases, CVT presents with signs and symptoms limited to those of increased ICP, thus mimicking IIH. The preferred study for the evaluation of suspected sinus thrombosis is MRI/MRV (see the above case, Headache and papilledema).

A diagnosis of CVT may be missed for several reasons. As noted above, the radiographic study may

be inadequate to demonstrate the lesion, or the timing of the investigation (very early or very late) may be responsible. In addition, the location of the clot influences its detectability. Thrombosis affecting the sagittal or straight sinus may pose a special challenge. Because there is no basis for comparison, the abnormal nature of the bright signal of the clot may not be appreciated. As in the identification of abnormalities involving the clivus and suprasellar cistern, it is important to be familiar with the normal appearance of these structures in order to identify abnormalities. Familiarity with the clinical findings that point to a disease process in these locations is the key to diagnosis.

Diagnosis: Superior sagittal sinus thrombosis

Tip: In a patient with unexplained increased intracranial pressure, particular attention should be paid to the superior sagittal sinus.

Vertical diplopia

Case: A 69-year-old retired coal miner noticed painless swelling around his left eye, and mild conjunctival injection. Four months later he developed similar swelling and redness of his right eye, and vertical diplopia. Examination five months after onset showed bilateral lid retraction with limitation of supraduction in each eye and an 18 diopter right hypertropia in primary position. An MRI of the orbits was read as normal but on closer inspection showed bilateral, symmetric enlargement of all extraocular muscles, consistent with Graves' disease (Figure 4.21).

Discussion: Disease processes in which the pathologic changes are bilateral and symmetric may be overlooked on imaging studies. Thyroid eye disease causes fusiform swelling of extraocular muscles that is usually bilateral and occasionally symmetric. The inferior rectus is the most commonly affected muscle, followed by the medial rectus. Occasionally all of the eye muscles are involved, as in the above patient. Contrast enhancement of the extraocular muscles is *not* pathologic, so this feature cannot

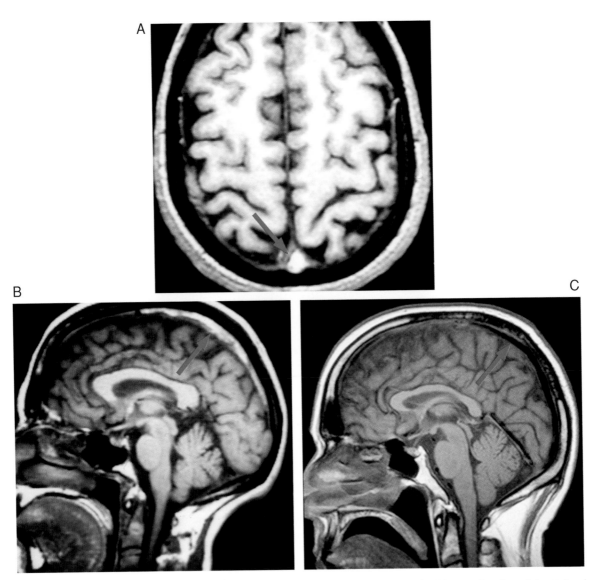

Figure 4.20 MRI of the above patient. (A) Axial and (B) sagittal non-contrast T1-weighted images show hyperintense signal within the superior sagittal sinus, characteristic of thrombosis (arrows). (C) Comparable sagittal view in a normal subject for comparison. Note the dark flow void of a normal superior sagittal sinus (arrow).

be used to identify the abnormality. Careful inspection for lid retraction, conjunctival injection and extraocular muscle dysfunction will usually point to the correct diagnosis, and attention to the scan can be directed accordingly.

Diagnosis: Symmetric Graves' disease

Tip: The diagnosis of thyroid eye disease may be missed when the radiographic changes are symmetric and mild.

A   B

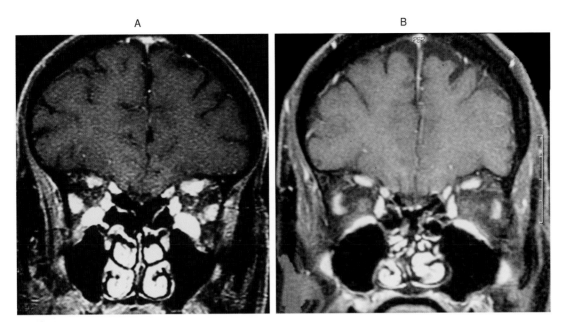

Figure 4.21 MRI of a 69-year-old retired coal miner with periorbital swelling and diplopia due to thyroid eye disease. (A) Coronal post-contrast fat-suppressed image shows mild symmetric enlargement of the extraocular muscles in both eyes. (B) Comparable view of the orbits of a normal subject for comparison. Note that contrast enhancement of the extraocular muscles is a normal feature.

FURTHER READING

Neuro-imaging

J. D. Trobe, S. S. Gebarski, Looking behind the eyes. The proper use of modern imaging. *Arch Ophthalmol*, **111** (1993), 1185–6.

R. J. Wolnitz, J. D. Trobe, W. T. Cornblath *et al.*, Common errors in the use of magnetic resonance imaging for neuro-ophthalmic diagnosis. *Surv Ophthalmol*, **45** (2000), 107–14.

Canalicular meningioma

C. L. Knight, W. F. Hoyt, C. B. Wilson, Syndrome of incipient prechiasmal optic nerve compression. *Arch Ophthalmol*, **87** (1972), 1–11.

S. Lessell, Current concepts in ophthalmology: optic neuropathies. *N Eng J Med*, **299** (1978), 533–6.

M. Pless, S. Lessell, Spontaneous visual improvement in orbital apex tumors. *Arch Ophthalmol*, **114** (1996), 704–6.

R. D. Tien, P. K. Chu, J. R. Hesselink, J. Szumowski, Intra and paraorbital lesions: value of fat suppression MR imaging with paramagnetic contrast enhancement. *Am J Roentgenol*, **156** (1991), 1059–67.

Cerebral venous thrombosis

R. H. Ayanzen, C. R. Bird, P. J. Keller *et al.*, Cerebral MR venography: normal anatomy and potential diagnostic pitfalls. *AJNR Am J Neuroradiol*, **21** (2000), 74–8.

V. Biousse, A. Ameri, M.-G. Bousser, Isolated intracranial hypertension as the only sign of cerebral venous thrombosis. *Neurology*, **53** (1999), 1537–42.

V. Biousse, M.-G. Bousser, Cerebral venous thrombosis. *Neurologist*, **5** (1999), 326–49.

D. I. Friedman, D. M. Jacobson, Diagnostic criteria for idiopathic intracranial hypertension. *Neurology*, **59** (2002), 1492–5.

A. Lin, R. Foroozan, H. V. Danesh-Meyer *et al.*, Occurrence of cerebral venous sinus thrombosis in patients with presumed idiopathic intracranial hypertension. *Ophthalmology*, **113** (2006), 2281–4.

V. Purvin, Venous occlusive disease. In N. R. Miller, N. J. Newman, V. Biousse, J. B. Kerrison, eds., *Walsh and Hoyt's Clinical Neuro-Ophthalmology*, 6th edn. Philadelphia:

Lippincott Williams and Wilkins, 2005, Vol. 2, Chapter 45, pp. 2427–65.

Horner syndrome and carotid dissection

V. Biousse, P. J. Touboul, J. D'Anglejan-Chatillon *et al.*, Ophthalmologic manifestations of internal carotid artery dissection. *Am J Ophthalmol*, **126** (1998), 565–s77.

J. Brown, R. Danielson, S. P. Donahue, Horner's syndrome in subadvential carotid artery dissection and the role of magnetic resonance angiography. *Am J Ophthalmol*, **6** (1995), 811–13.

K. B. Digre, W. R. Smoker, P. Johnston *et al.*, Selective MR imaging approach for evaluation of patients with Horner's syndrome. *Am J Neuroradiol*, **13** (1992), 223–7.

W. F. Maloney, B. R. Younge, N. J. Moyer, Evaluation of the causes and accuracy of pharmacologic localization in Horner's syndrome. *Am J Ophthalmol*, **90** (1980), 394–402.

B. Mokri, Traumatic and spontaneous extracranial internal carotid artery dissection: early diagnosis and management. *J Neurol*, **237** (1990), 356–61.

Pituitary apoplexy

V. Biousse, N. J. Newman, N. M. Oyesiku, Precipitating factors in pituitary apoplexy. *J Neurol Neurosurg Psychiatr*, **71** (2001), 542–5.

W. Bonicki, A. Kasperlik-Zaluska, W. Koszewski, W. Zgliczyński, J. Wislawski, Pituitary apoplexy: endocrine, surgical and oncological emergency. Incidence, clinical course and treatment with reference to 799 cases of pituitary adenomas. *Acta Neurochir*, **120** (1993), 118–22.

N. J. David, Pituitary apoplexy goes to the bar: litigation for delayed diagnosis, deficient vision, and death. *J Neuroophthalmol*, **26** (2006), 128–33.

S. Milazzo, P. Toussaint, F. Proust, G. Touzet, D. Malthieu, Ophthalmologic aspects of pituitary apoplexy. *Eur J Ophthalmol*, **6** (1996), 69–73.

Chronic sixth nerve palsy

J. Currie, J. H. Lubin, S. Lessell, Chronic isolated abducens paresis from tumors at the base of the brain. *Arch Neurol*, **40** (1983), 226–9.

J. R. Keane, Bilateral sixth nerve palsy. Analysis of 125 cases. *Arch Neurol*, **33** (1976), 681–3.

F. Kimura, K. S. Kim, H. Friedman, E. J. Russell, R. Breit, MR imaging of the normal and abnormal clivus. *AJNR Am J Neuroradiol*, **11** (1990), 1015–21.

P. J. Savino, J. K. Hilliker, G. H. Casell, N. J. Schatz, Chronic sixth nerve palsies: are they really harbingers of serious intracranial disease? *Arch Ophthalmol*, **100** (1982), 1442–4.

5

Incidental findings (seeing but not believing)

Certain signs and symptoms are seen frequently as a normal variant in some individuals but may also signify illness in others. An example of this is the decreased sense of smell that may be normal in a long-term smoker but is also a classic symptom of a subfrontal meningioma. Similarly, facial asymmetry may be written off as a normal congenital variant but can also be a subtle sign of mild seventh nerve paresis from a growing brainstem tumor. Deciding when a sign or symptom should be pursued and when it should be ignored is a valuable clinical skill. This is also true when interpreting radiographic findings. Certain scan abnormalities that may occur in some individuals as a normal variant or an incidental finding (sometimes termed an "incidentaloma") may be a sign of a disease process in others. In this section we look at a few such examples. In each case, it is the responsibility of the clinician to correlate the scan finding with the clinical information in order to appreciate its diagnostic significance. Part of this process should include personally reviewing the scan in the context of the clinical abnormalities, rather than relying on a written radiographic report.

Empty sella

Case: A 36-year-old homemaker sought medical attention because of intermittent horizontal diplopia. She had gained weight following each of her three pregnancies and had a long history of chronic daily headaches but was otherwise healthy.

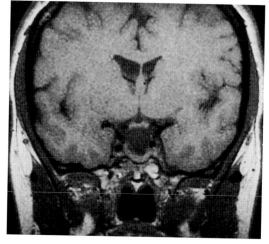

Figure 5.1 Empty sella. Coronal non-contrast T1-weighted MRI of a 36-year-old homemaker with IIH shows enlargement of the sella turcica and downward flattening of the pituitary gland.

Examination showed mild fullness of the optic discs with normal optic nerve function and normal ocular motility. A brain MRI was unremarkable except for an enlarged and "empty" sella, reported as a normal variant (Figure 5.1). She was treated with a series of medications for muscle contraction headaches and then for migraine without much success. Eventually, a lumbar puncture was performed which demonstrated elevated intracranial pressure (ICP) of 300 mm of water with normal cerebrospinal fluid constituents, leading to a diagnosis of idiopathic intracranial hypertension (IIH).

Discussion: An enlarged sella without associated enlargement of the pituitary gland sometimes occurs following treatment of a pituitary tumor or after pituitary apoplexy and, in this context, is referred to as *"secondary" empty sella syndrome.* In contrast, patients with this finding and no prior history of pituitary enlargement are said to have *"primary" empty sella syndrome.* This radiographic finding may occur as a normal variant, reportedly seen in up to 20% of normal individuals, or it may be a sign of long-standing increased ICP.

Although the original definition of IIH stipulates that radiographic studies must be normal, minor abnormalities are in fact commonly seen, particularly on MR rather than CT scans. A study examining the MRI findings in a group of 20 patients with idiopathic intracranial hypertension found that subtle radiographic abnormalities indicative of increased ICP were common in IIH. Flattening of the posterior globe was seen in 80% of patients, an empty sella in 70% and expansion of the perioptic spaces in 45% (Figure 5.2A and B). In addition, papilledema was frequently visible, appearing as enhancement of the prelaminar optic nerve in 50% and as intraocular protrusion of the optic nerve in 30% (Figure 5.2C). A small degree of cerebellar tonsillar descent is also seen in some patients with chronically increased ICP.

Low cerebellar tonsils

Case: A 27-year-old woman with a history of chronic headaches experienced new onset of blurred vision, intermittent horizontal diplopia and occasional paresthesias in her arms and legs. Her examination revealed normal visual function and fundus appearance. She had a comitant esophoria that broke down easily to an esotropia but no ductional deficit and no saccadic slowing. She had a little difficulty with tandem gait and an otherwise normal neurologic examination. Demyelinating disease was suspected and an MR scan was obtained (Figure 5.3). The scan showed no white-matter lesions although the official report did mention mild protrusion of the cerebellar tonsils through the foramen magnum. The patient's physician noted this on the report but considered it to be an incidental finding. The patient was reassured that there was no sign of multiple sclerosis.

Discussion: A comitant esodeviation without a ductional deficit is most often due to congenital esotropia in children, and to decompensation of a pre-existing esophoria when encountered in adults. Less commonly, comitant esotropia is due to acquired disease, usually related to increased ICP or involving the posterior fossa. Specific causes

A   B   C

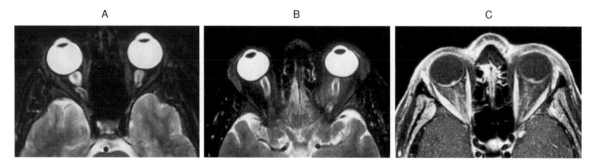

Figure 5.2 Radiographic abnormalities commonly seen in increased intracranial pressure. (A) Axial fat-suppressed T2-weighted MRI shows expansion of the perioptic spaces. (B) Similar study of a different patient shows flattening of the posterior globe, more on the right than the left, due to pressure from expanded perioptic spaces. (C) Bilateral papilledema appears as nodular enhancement of the optic nerve heads on this axial post-contrast fat-suppressed T1-weighted MRI.

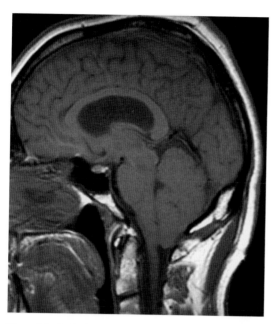

Figure 5.3 Sagittal non-contrast T1-weighted MRI in the above patient shows mild descent of the cerebellar tonsils below the foramen magnum. Note very mild compression of the lower brainstem.

include brainstem and cerebellar tumors, strokes, degenerative diseases and hind-brain anomalies such as the Chiari malformation (see Chapter 7, Bouncing vision). Comitant esotropia associated with Chiari I malformation is believed to be related to a disturbance in the vergence mechanism rather than to dysfunction of the sixth nerves. In nearly all cases, it is accompanied by other symptoms and signs of hindbrain overcrowding. In light of the patient's clinical findings, the tonsillar descent was re-interpreted as a symptomatic Chiari I malformation. Following sub-occipital decompression, her headaches and diplopia resolved, however intermittent paresthesias persisted.

Sphenoid sinus mucocele

Case: A 78-year-old retired teacher had a four-month history of progressive horizontal diplopia. Initially her double vision occurred only on extreme

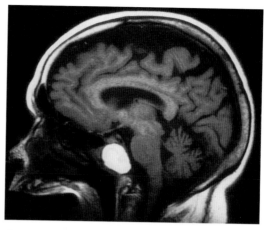

Figure 5.4 Sagittal non-contrast T1-weighted MRI in 78-year-old woman with a progressive sixth nerve palsy shows a large sphenoid sinus mucocele.

right gaze but over time it came to involve primary position as well, first at distance and then at near. Examination showed a partial right sixth nerve palsy and was otherwise unrevealing. An MR scan was reportedly normal except for a mucocele in the sphenoid sinus, which was assumed to be an incidental finding. Results of additional laboratory testing and a lumbar puncture were non-diagnostic and she was therefore referred for neuro-ophthalmic consultation. Review of her outside scan showed a large, round hyperintensity in the sphenoid sinus consistent with a mucocele. The mass was noted to extend posteriorly, eroding through to the back of the clivus where it was believed to be compromising the sixth nerve (Figure 5.4). She underwent transphenoidal excision of the lesion, histopathologically confirmed as a mucocele, and over the weeks following surgery her diplopia and sixth nerve palsy resolved completely.

Discussion: Sinus disease is so common in the normal population that it is frequently encountered on a radiologic study obtained for another purpose and dismissed as an incidental finding. For example, a study examining the incidence of sinus disease in a series of patients with optic neuritis found no difference compared to a group of healthy controls (about 13% in each group). In the above case, however, the mucocele was not incidental. Its significance could be appreciated when the scan appearance was correlated with the clinical findings. The mucocele had grown posteriorly into the pathway of the sixth nerve as it ascends the clivus.

Because sinus disease is so common in certain geographic areas, it is important to have some guidelines to help decide when it has clinical significance. Particular attention should be given to sinus disease when there is bony erosion with extension into neighboring soft tissues. Sinusitis that invades the orbit can mimic any form of the idiopathic orbital inflammatory syndrome. Sinusitis that seeds the cavernous sinus can result in a life-threatening cavernous sinus thrombosis. In some cases, the patient demographics should arouse suspicion. For example, poorly controlled diabetics, especially those in ketoacidosis, immunosuppressed individuals, patients with hematologic malignancies and those on hemodialysis are especially susceptible to fungal sinusitis. A patient with any of these risk factors who develops an acute orbital inflammatory syndrome with evidence of paranasal sinusitis should be investigated promptly for mucormycosis, as this rapidly invasive infection has a high mortality rate. Such patients are also prone to aspergillosis, which may similarly spread from the adjacent sinuses into the orbit where it may present as a mass lesion.

Dolichoectatic basilar artery

Case: A 70-year-old retired radiologist had a two-year history of painless horizontal diplopia. At first, his double vision had been intermittent but was now constant and caused him to feel off balance while walking. He reported no other neurologic or systemic symptoms. Past medical history included hypertension, coronary artery disease and a hemispheric TIA due to carotid stenosis, treated with endarterectomy several years earlier. His neurologic status had been stable since then. On examination, there was a moderate right abduction deficit

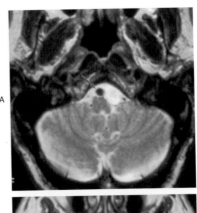

A

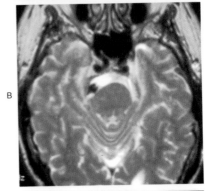

B

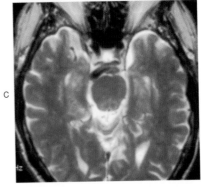

C

Figure 5.5 MRI in the above patient with a painless, chronic right sixth nerve palsy. This sequence of axial T2-weighted images shows the course of the basilar artery. (A) The basilar artery, seen here as a low-intensity signal void (arrow) is positioned in the midline at the ventral medulla. (B) At the pontine level, the basilar artery is slightly enlarged and is clearly shifted to the right where it compresses and flattens the ventral aspect of the pons. (C) At the midbrain, the basilar artery is seen at an oblique angle as it redirects its course back toward the midline.

causing an esotropia that worsened on right gaze. Abduction saccades in the right eye were slow. The remainder of his examination was unremarkable and a Tensilon (edrophonium chloride) test was negative.

A CBC, ESR, CRP, acetylcholine receptor antibodies and antiGQ1b antibodies were normal. An MRI of brain and orbits was interpreted as normal although the radiologist's report noted tortuosity of the basilar artery. A lumbar puncture showed a normal opening pressure and CSF constituents. In light of the negative evaluation and progressive cranial nerve palsy, the patient was referred for neuro-ophthalmic consultation.

A critical review of the MR scan, in the context of the patient's clinical findings, revealed that the ectatic and tortuous basilar artery was distorting the ventral surface of the pons, particularly on the right side at the exit zone of the sixth nerve (Figure 5.5). Based on a combination of the clinical and radiographic features, a diagnosis of dolichoectatic com-

pression of the sixth nerve was made. His esotropia progressed slightly over the next eight months then stabilized for the next three years. The patient was managed symptomatically with prisms and a follow-up MRI was unchanged.

Discussion: Dolichoectasia describes abnormal elongation, distention and tortuosity of blood vessels. The prevalence of intracranial dolichoectasia is estimated at 0.06 to 5.8%, most frequently involving the vertebrobasilar system in which the anomaly is sometimes referred to as a fusiform aneurysm of the basilar artery. The pathogenesis of dolichoectasia is not completely understood but the condition is strongly associated with arteriosclerosis and chronic hypertension. Histopathologically, there is diffuse loss of elastic tissue and atrophy of smooth muscle cells, structures which normally protect the arterial wall from the expansile effects of high systolic pressure.

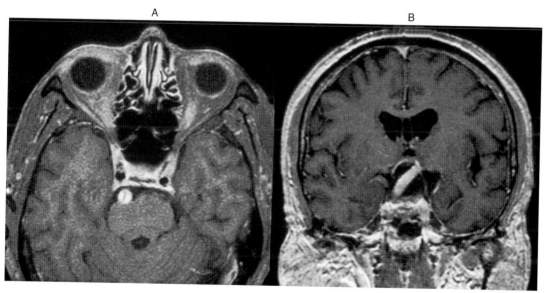

Figure 5.6 Another example of vertebrobasilar artery dolichoectasia. This patient had a chronic right sixth nerve palsy and a mild bitemporal visual field defect. (A) Axial post-contrast fat-suppressed T1-weighted MR image shows compression and distortion of the ventral pons by the basilar artery. (B) The coronal image shows the ectatic basilar artery extending upward into the suprasellar cistern, causing chiasmal compression.

The radiographic appearance and clinical presentation of vertebrobasilar dolichoectasia are variable. In some patients, it is clinically silent and represents an incidental radiographic finding. In other cases, such tortuosity produces neurologic dysfunction by a variety of mechanisms. There may be direct compression of the brainstem or cranial nerves, stroke-like events related to thrombosis, microembolization or hemodynamic disturbance, and occasionally hydrocephalus. A causal relationship between a particular clinical finding and this radiologic anomaly should be made only after exclusion of other possible causes. MRI combined with MRA is the optimal imaging technique for evaluating the anatomical relationship between vessels and neural structures, particularly vascular compression of cranial nerves. Isolated cranial nerve involvement, as in the patient described above, may be the sole manifestation of vertebrobasilar dolichoectasia, and any cranial nerve except the olfactory nerve is susceptible (Figure 5.6).

Management of patients with neurologic manifestations related to vertebrobasilar dolichoectasia is generally conservative. Most patients do not progress beyond an isolated cranial neuropathy and are treated with observation, prisms and occasionally strabismus surgery.

FURTHER READING

Pseudotumor cerebri syndrome

M. C. Brodsky, M. Vaphiades, Magnetic resonance imaging in pseudotumor cerebri. *Ophthalmology*, **105** (1998), 1686–93.

K. M. Foley, J. B. Posner, Does pseudotumor cerebri cause the empty sella syndrome? *Neurology*, **25** (1975), 565–9.

Chiari malformation

V. Biousse, N. J. Newman, S. H. Petermann, S. R. Lambert, Isolated comitant esotropia and Chiari I malformation. *Am J Ophthalmol*, **130** (2000), 216–20.

S. J. Hentschel, K. G. Yen, F. F. Lang, Chiari I malformation and acute acquired comitant esotropia: case report and review of the literature. *J Neurosurg*, **102** (2005), 407–12.

T. H. Milhorat, M. W. Chou, E. M. Trinidad *et al.*, Chiari I malformation redefined: clinical and radiographic findings for 364 symptomatic patients. *Neurosurgery*, **44** (1999), 1005–17.

Sphenoid sinus mucocele

M. Ada, A. Kaytaz, K. Tuskan, M. G. Guvenc, H. Silcuk, Isolated sphenoid sinusitis presenting with unilateral VIth nerve palsy. *International J Ped Otorhinolaryngol*, **68** (2004), 507–10.

Dolichoectatic basilar artery

N. Goldenberg-Cohen, N. R. Miller, Noninvasive neuroimaging of basilar artery dolichoectasia in a patient with an isolated abducens nerve paresis. *Am J Ophthalmol*, **137** (2004), 365–7.

S. G. Passero, S. Rossi, Natural history of vertebrobasilar dolichoectasia. *Neurology*, **70**, (2008), 66–72.

W. R. K. Smoker. J. J. Corbett, L. R. Gentry *et al.*, High-resolution computed tomography of the basilar artery: 2. Vertebrobasilar dolichoectasia: clinical-pathologic correlation and review. *AJNR*, **7** (1986), 61–72.

6

Failure of pattern recognition

Some neuro-ophthalmic signs and symptoms are non-specific, produced by a variety of disease processes in more than one location within the neuraxis. In certain cases, however, a particular combination of findings can only be due to a disease process in one place. For example, the combination of an ipsilateral optic neuropathy and contralateral superior temporal defect indicates a lesion at the junction of the optic nerve and chiasm, referred to as a "junctional scotoma". So-called "crossed brainstem syndromes" in which there is an ipsilateral cranial neuropathy and contralateral long tract deficit are another such example. Similarly, the presence of an ipsilateral Horner syndrome and contralateral fourth nerve palsy is exquisitely localizing to an area in the midbrain lateral to the cerebral aqueduct, involving the descending sympathetic fibers and the fascicles from the trochlear nucleus prior to their decussation. In some of these conditions, the responsible lesion is small or otherwise subtle, and in these cases the clinical findings are particularly valuable for pointing to the correct diagnosis. This chapter consists of several such examples in which accurate diagnosis depends on familiarity with these patterns.

Painful ophthalmoplegia

Case: A 35-year-old construction worker developed pain behind the left eye radiating up to the brow and vertex on that side. Several days later he experienced oblique diplopia and drooping of the left upper lid that worsened over several days. Examination three weeks after onset showed complete left upper lid ptosis and marked external ophthalmoplegia of the left eye, including absence of incyclotorsion on attempted downgaze (Figure 6.1). There was mild anisocoria, left pupil smaller than the right, that was best seen in dim illumination; but both pupils reacted briskly to light stimulation. Afferent visual function was normal. There was decreased sensation to pain and temperature in the distribution of the ophthalmic division of the left trigeminal nerve, as well as a decreased corneal reflex on that side. An MRI was reportedly normal (Figure 6.2), as were the results of a number of blood tests, urinalysis, tuberculosis skin test and chest radiograph.

Where is this patient's lesion?

This patient presented with painful unilateral ophthalmoplegia. His examination indicated dysfunction of cranial nerves three, four, six, the ophthalmic branch of five, and the oculosympathetics on the left side. This constellation of findings is exquisitely localizing to the region of the cavernous sinus and superior orbital fissure. Though anatomically distinct spaces, there is not a way to distinguish clinically between a lesion of the cavernous sinus and one in the superior orbital fissure, and therefore the constellation of findings that results from a lesion in this area is sometimes referred to as the *"sphenocavernous syndrome"*. Because so many nerves pass through so small a space, even a very small lesion in this area can produce multiple cranial nerve deficits.

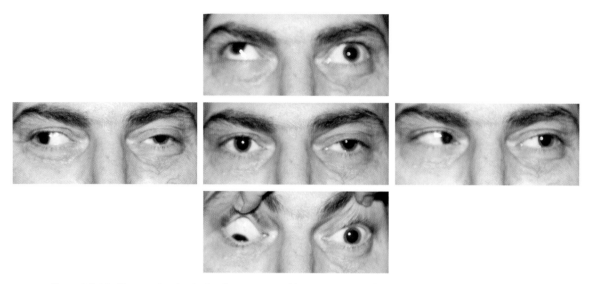

Figure 6.1 Motility examination in the above 35-year-old construction worker with acute painful ophthalmoplegia. There is moderate left upper lid ptosis and marked limitation of left eye movements in all directions. (The pupils are pharmacologically dilated.)

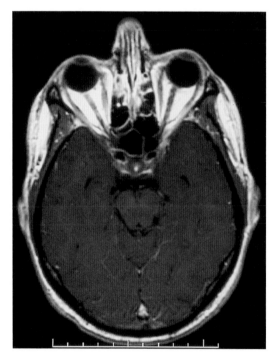

Figure 6.2 MRI of the same patient. This axial post-contrast T1-weighted image was read as normal.

Careful inspection of this patient's MRI disclosed an abnormal hyperintensity within the superior orbital fissure on post-contrast T1-weighted images (Figure 6.3). Despite the severity of this patient's clinical findings, the radiographic abnormality was surprisingly subtle. Tests for specific systemic inflammatory disorders were unrevealing and a presumptive diagnosis of Tolosa Hunt syndrome was made. He was treated with high-dose oral prednisone (80 mg per day), which brought prompt relief of his pain. Re-examination one month later showed dramatic improvement of ocular motility with normal trigeminal sensation. He continued a slow taper of his steroids over the next several months, with eventual resolution of his clinical deficits and radiographic abnormality.

Discussion: Tolosa Hunt syndrome is an idiopathic granulomatous inflammatory process involving the area of the cavernous sinus and superior orbital fissure, causing painful ophthalmoplegia. There are no serologic markers for this condition and it is rarely necessary or appropriate to biopsy these structures,

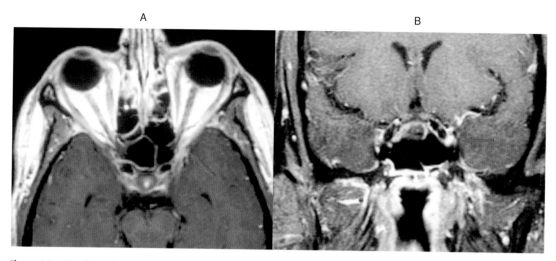

Figure 6.3 MRI of the above patient with a left spheno-cavernous syndrome. (A) Close-up view of the axial image shown in Figure 6.2 reveals a small area of enhancement within the left superior orbital fissure (arrow). (B) Coronal post-contrast fat-suppressed T1-weighted image confirms the abnormality (arrow).

Table 6.1 International Headache Society criteria for the diagnosis of Tolosa Hunt syndrome (*Cephalalgia,* **24** Suppl 1 (2004))

1. One or more episodes of unilateral orbital pain lasting weeks if untreated
2. Paralysis of one or more cranial nerves three, four, six and/or demonstration of granuloma by MRI or biopsy
3. Paresis coincides with onset of pain or follows it within two weeks
4. Pain and paresis resolve within 72 hours when treated adequately with steroids
5. Other causes have been excluded by appropriate investigations

and thus the diagnosis is typically a clinical one (see Table 6.1).

Tolosa Hunt syndrome (THS) typically presents with acute onset of periorbital or hemi-cranial pain associated with numbness or paresthesias if the trigeminal nerve is involved. In addition, there is ipsilateral paralysis of one or more ocular motor cranial nerves and Horner syndrome in varying combination. In up to 20% of cases the inflammation extends anteriorly to produce optic nerve dysfunction. Involvement of the seventh nerve is an uncommon manifestation. It is important to recognize that this constellation of findings simply localizes a lesion to the cavernous sinus/superior orbital fissure region and is not specific for THS. The list of diseases that can affect the parasellar region is broad, and a diagnosis of Tolosa Hunt syndrome is one of exclusion after other causes have been ruled out (see Table 6.2).

MR imaging is often abnormal in patients with THS. The contents of the cavernous sinus are usually best assessed by inspection of thin section T1-weighted post-contrast views in the coronal plane. In most cases of THS there is enlargement and increased enhancement of the cavernous sinus. When mild, this may appear as loss of the normal concavity of the lateral wall as seen on both coronal and axial images (Figure 6.4). There may also be enhancement of the adjacent dural wall and abnormal soft tissue surrounding and narrowing the cavernous internal carotid artery. In occasional cases there is extension of this abnormal soft tissue into the orbital apex, sphenoid sinus or floor of the middle cranial fossa. However it is important to be aware that in some cases even high quality imaging may be normal. In other cases, a radiographic

Table 6.2 Etiologies of cavernous sinus syndrome

Tumors
  meningioma
  lymphoma
  nasopharyngeal carcinoma
  pituitary tumor
  metastatic disease
Vascular abnormalities
  internal carotid artery aneurysm
  carotid or dural fistula
  cavernous sinus fistula
Inflammatory disorders
  sarcoidosis
  syphilis
  tuberculosis
  Wegener's granulomatosis
  fungal disease (e.g. aspergillosis)

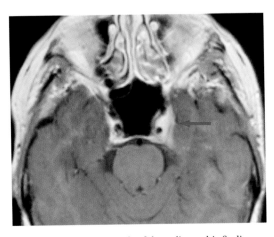

Figure 6.4 Another example of the radiographic findings in a cavernous sinus syndrome. Axial post-contrast T1-weighted MR image of a 60-year-old woman with a cavernous sinus meningioma shows expansion of the left cavernous sinus producing loss of the usual concavity seen on the normal right side (arrow). This is an early (though non-specific) sign of cavernous sinus disease.

abnormality is present but wrongly attributed to normal asymmetry of venous flow within the cavernous sinuses.

The radiographic abnormalities associated with THS are non-specific and can also be seen in other inflammatory conditions and with a variety of neoplasms including meningioma, lymphoma and metastatic tumors. There are no established MRI criteria for the diagnosis of THS. In addition to high-quality imaging, investigations should include sero-logic tests for inflammatory disorders (complete blood count (CBC), erythrocyte sedimentation rate (ESR), angiotensin converting enzyme (ACE), flu-orescent treponemal antibody (FTA) and antineu-trophilic cytoplasmic antibodies), tests for tuberculosis (TB skin test and chest radiograph), urinalysis and lumbar puncture. Referral to an otolaryngologist should be considered to further investigate for nasopharyngeal tumor or fungal disease. In some cases, a biopsy of the nasopharynx is appropriate, even in the absence of abnormalities on the mirror examination.

The etiology of the inflammatory process in THS is unknown. As in other forms of idiopathic inflammation, corticosteroids are the mainstay of treatment. Resolution of pain within 24–48 hours of initiation of steroids is characteristic but non-specific, as other inflammatory and even neoplastic processes involving the cavernous sinus may also be dramatically steroid-responsive.

Diagnosis: Tolosa Hunt syndrome

Tip: The clinical features of a cavernous sinus/superior orbital fissure syndrome are highly localizing, but radiographic abnormalities are easily overlooked.

Painful ophthalmoplegia and visual loss

Case: A 58-year-old homemaker with a past history of breast cancer experienced left-sided headaches followed one month later by vertical diplopia. Examination at that time showed slight left upper lid ptosis and a mild left hypotropia with normal afferent visual function. Over the next few weeks, left eye movements became increasingly limited and she developed dimming of vision in that eye. A CT scan was reportedly normal. Neuro-ophthalmic examination two months after onset of symptoms showed complete ophthalmoplegia of the left eye and a left optic neuropathy. Visual acuity was 20/80 OS with

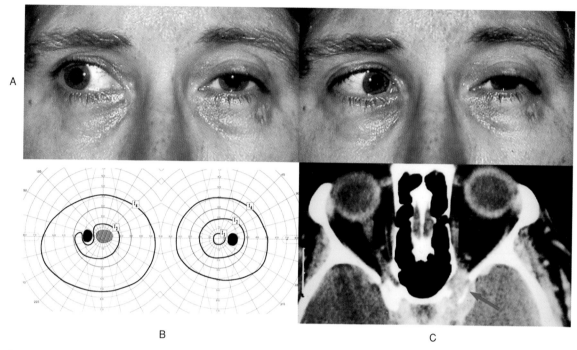

Figure 6.5 Examination findings in the above patient with a two-month history of progressive left ophthalmoplegia and optic neuropathy. (A) The left lid is ptotic and there is marked limitation of both adduction and abduction. (B) Goldmann perimetry shows a small but dense central scotoma OS. (C) Axial post-contrast CT image reveals an enhancing mass eroding the left anterior clinoid, encroaching on the superior orbital fissure and extending into the orbital apex (arrow).

poor color vision and a central scotoma (Figure 6.5A and B). All findings in the right eye were normal.

Based on the clinical findings, where is the lesion?

Based on the clinical features, a lesion at the orbital apex was suspected. A new CT scan showed a lesion at the left superior orbital fissure extending into the orbital apex (Figure 6.5C).

The clinical and radiographic findings were most consistent with metastatic disease. A nuclear bone scan revealed increased uptake in the thoracic and lumbar spine and in several ribs, confirming widespread metastatic disease beyond the orbit. She received radiation therapy to the left orbital apex and was started on chemotherapy. Just as radiation was begun she suffered additional loss of vision in

the left eye due to central retinal artery occlusion. Following completion of radiation, her ocular motility improved but vision in that eye failed to recover.

Discussion: Involvement of the ocular motor nerves as they enter the orbit through the superior fissure accompanied by optic neuropathy comprises the *orbital apex syndrome*. Clinical findings are the same as those seen in the spheno-cavernous syndrome with the addition of ipsilateral visual loss and variable proptosis. In its complete form there is paralysis of all eye movements, oculosympathetic palsy and sensory loss and/or pain in the distribution of the first division of the trigeminal nerve, as well as optic neuropathy. Incomplete forms are common, however, and should be recognizable to the clinician. Because of the close proximity of the cavernous sinus, superior orbital fissure and orbital apex, any pathologic process can begin in one of these regions and then spread to involve neighboring structures, as in the above case. The patient's initial diplopia was due to tumor in the superior orbital fissure which subsequently extended into the orbital apex producing optic nerve compression.

Disease processes that cause the orbital apex syndrome include primary and metastatic orbital neoplasms, tumors invading the orbit from adjacent structures (sinuses, nasopharynx and sphenoid wing), ischemia and a variety of inflammatory disorders such as mucormycosis, aspergillosis and herpes zoster. In most cases of orbital disease due to any of these mechanisms, the presence of orbital signs, particularly proptosis, helps to localize the disease process. At the orbital apex, however, there is so little extra room that even a small mass can produce significant visual loss *in the absence of proptosis*. In addition, this area is notoriously difficult to visualize on radiographic studies. MRI is superior to CT in the evaluation of soft tissue lesions in the posterior orbit, but even with a high quality scan the responsible abnormality may difficult to appreciate, particularly at low field or if fat suppression is not used. Familiarity with the pattern of clinical findings in this syndrome should aid in its recognition.

Diagnosis: Orbital apex syndrome

Tip: The combination of ipsilateral ophthalmoplegia and optic neuropathy is a distinctive pattern indicating a lesion at the orbital apex.

Painless diplopia

Case: This 14-year-old girl had a six-month history of double vision on left gaze, unassociated with headache or eye pain. She had been generally healthy and reported no prior history of head trauma, diplopia or ptosis. On examination, eye movements were full except for moderate limitation of adduction in the right eye. The right pupil was 2 mm larger than the left pupil and its direct and consensual response to light stimulation was a bit sluggish. The eyelids were aligned in primary position but changed on gaze to either side (Figure 6.6). There were no other focal neurologic deficits. CT and MRI were read as normal.

What is this motility pattern, and what does it tell you about the mechanism of the patient's diplopia?

This patient exhibits lid retraction on adduction, which represents a synkinesis between third nerve neurons. This is an example of third nerve misdirection, and it indicates mechanical damage to the peripheral oculomotor nerve. Her radiographic studies were critically re-evaluated in light of this rather subtle finding, and a very small mass was identified within the right cavernous sinus (Figure 6.7). This lesion was compatible with either a meningioma or schwannoma and she was managed expectantly. Over the next few years her third nerve palsy showed slow additional progression.

Discussion: Third nerve misdirection, also termed *aberrant regeneration* or *oculomotor synkinesis*,

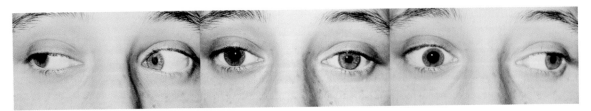

Figure 6.6 Eye movements in a 14-year-old girl with a six-month history of diplopia. Adduction of the right eye is moderately limited and the right pupil is enlarged. Note that the lids are symmetric in primary gaze but the right lid droops on right gaze and elevates on left gaze.

A   B

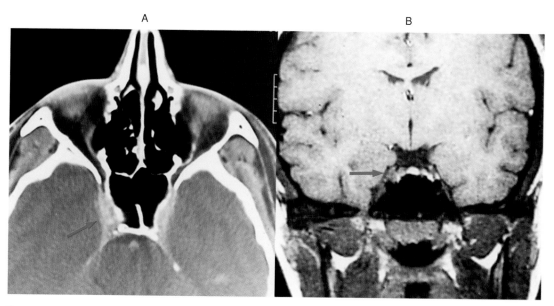

Figure 6.7 Radiographic studies in the above 14-year-old girl with a right cavernous sinus tumor. (A) Axial post-contrast CT shows subtle expansion of the right cavernous sinus. Note loss of the normal concave shape of the lateral wall (arrow), often the earliest sign of cavernous sinus disease. (B) Coronal non-contrast T1-weighted MRI shows subtle homogeneous soft-tissue density within the right cavernous sinus (arrow).

occurs when stimulation of one branch of the third nerve results in co-activation of another third nerve branch. The various patterns of misdirection can be predicted by "mixing and matching" any two third nerve muscles. The most commonly recognized form of oculomotor synkinesis is lid retraction on adduction (as seen in this patient) or on downgaze (Figure 6.8). When third nerve misdirection involves the pupil, there is a poor response to light stimulation but constriction on attempted adduction or vertical gaze. While this occurs more commonly than aberrant lid innervation, it is technically more difficult to detect, often requiring the use of a slit-lamp. In any of its forms, third nerve misdirection is easy to overlook because its demonstration requires doing one thing while watching another, for instance having the patient look to the side but observing the lids. In a patient with a third nerve palsy, particularly one in which the diagnosis is in question, it is important to specifically look for

misdirection after assessing range of motion, pupillary responses and lid position and function.

The mechanism underlying oculomotor synkinesis is misdirection of regenerating axons with subsequent faulty reinnervation of target muscles. The significance of this phenomenon is that it indicates mechanical damage to third nerve axons. This kind of injury is common after aneurysmal rupture or head trauma, and in this setting is sometimes referred to as "secondary" aberrant regeneration. In contrast, "primary" aberrant regeneration indicates the presence of oculomotor synkinesis without a previous history of third nerve palsy. Patients who present with primary misdirection almost always harbor a compressive lesion, typically an intracavernous carotid aneurysm or a meningioma, as in the case under discussion. Thus, the finding of lid retraction on adduction in this patient strongly indicated the presence of an occult structural lesion in contact with the third nerve, which was ultimately

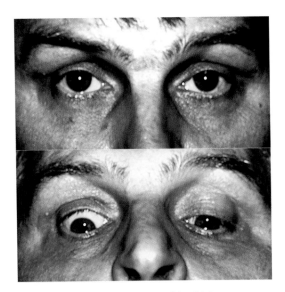

Figure 6.8 Aberrant regeneration of the third nerve following trauma. Four months after transtentorial herniation due to a subdural hematoma, this patient exhibits lid retraction on downgaze. This distinctive finding was the only residual sign of his previous third nerve palsy.

demonstrated on her MR scan. Recognition of this particular pattern of ocular motor dysfunction can be the key to the detection of small or subtle lesions.

Diagnosis: Oculomotor nerve palsy with aberrant regeneration

Tip: For practical purposes, oculomotor synkinesis always indicates *mechanical* damage to the third nerve. The presence of oculomotor synkinesis without a previous history of acute third nerve palsy indicates a compressive lesion.

Right-sided visual field loss

Case: A 67-year-old, hypertensive, diabetic homemaker experienced sudden onset of difficulty seeing to the right. A brain MRI showed a number of scattered hyperintensities on T2-weighted images, which were interpreted as non-specific small vessel disease (Figure 6.9A). She was told that her scan had

ruled out a stroke. Subsequent neuro-ophthalmic examination included Goldmann visual fields that showed a right homonymous sectoranopia (Figure 6.9B).

What is the significance of this visual field pattern? Does it help to illuminate the findings on her MRI?

This unusual wedge-shaped homonymous defect with its apex pointing to fixation is termed a *homonymous horizontal sectoranopia*. It constitutes a distinctive pattern of field loss produced by a vascular injury to the *lateral geniculate body*. Although the patient's MRI shows a number of white matter lesions consistent with small vessel disease, the one in the left lateral geniculate body represents an acute infarct, which was the cause of her visual loss.

Discussion: Axons from the retinal ganglion cells synapse in the lateral geniculate body (LGB) to form the geniculocalcarine radiations. This nucleus is a cap-like structure that is located in the posterior aspect of the thalamus, below and lateral to the pulvinar and above the lateral recess of the ambient cistern (Figure 6.10A). The dorsal region of the nucleus subserves macular function, the lateral and medial aspects subserve the superior and the inferior fields respectively (Figure 6.10B). The LGB has a dual blood supply: the lateral choroidal artery (branch of the posterior cerebral artery) supplies the macular zone, whereas the anterior choroidal artery (a branch of the internal carotid artery) supplies the lateral and medial horns. As a consequence of this anatomic arrangement, occlusion of either vessel can produce a distinctive visual field pattern. Infarction in the territory of the lateral choroidal artery results in a congruous, wedge-shaped defect termed a *"horizontal sectoranopia"*, as in the above case. Occlusion of the anterior choroidal artery produces a complementary pattern, termed a *"quadruple sectoranopia"* (Figure 6.11).

Despite rare case reports of horizontal sectoranopia due to a lesion of the geniculocalcarine

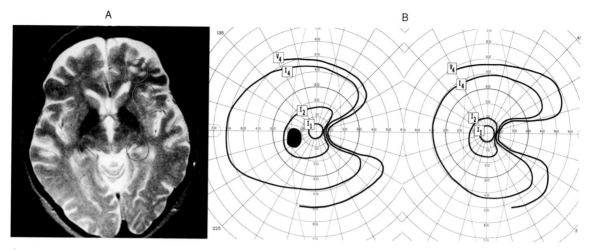

Figure 6.9 (A) Axial T2-weighted MR image reveals a few small areas of white matter hyperintensity, interpreted as representing small vessel disease (circles). (B) Goldmann perimetry shows a right congruous homonymous wedge-shaped defect extending toward fixation.

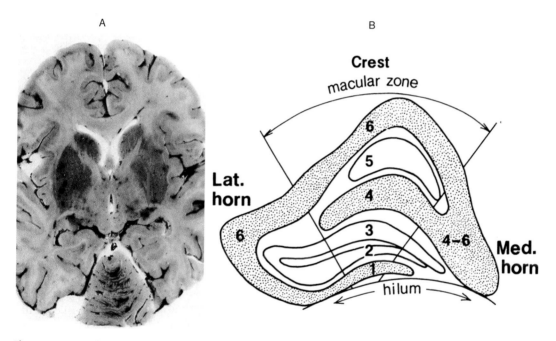

Figure 6.10 Lateral geniculate anatomy. (A) Axial brain slice shows the location of the lateral geniculate body (arrow). (From J. C. Horton, K. Landau, R. Maeder, *et al.*, Magnetic resonance imaging of the human lateral geniculate body. *Arch Neurol*, **47** (1990), 1201–6, with permission.) (B) Schematic drawing of a coronal section through the LGB viewed from its posterior aspect, illustrating its topographic organization. There are six laminae corresponding to different retinal ganglion cell inputs. Three laminae (layer two, three, and five – white areas) receive input from ipsilateral retinal ganglion cells, and three laminae (stippled layers one, four, and six) receive input from contralateral retinal ganglion cells. (From *Walsh and Hoyt's Clinical Neuro-Ophthalmology*, 5th edn. N. R. Miller, N. J. Newman, eds. Philadelphia: Lippincott Williams and Wilkins, 1998, Vol. 1, Chapter 5, p. 106, with permission.)

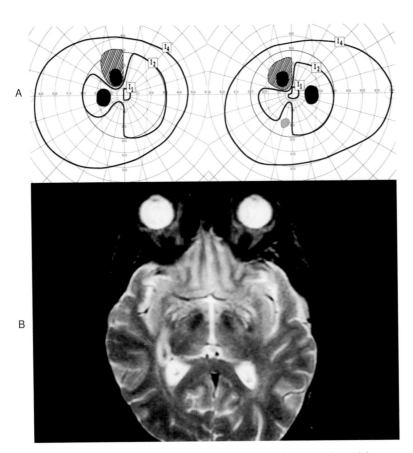

Figure 6.11 Example of a quadruple sectoranopia due to right anterior choroidal artery occlusion. (A) There is homonymous field loss involving the upper and lower quadrants but sparing central fibers. (B) Axial FLAIR MR image demonstrates the corresponding right LGB stroke (arrow).

radiations rather than the LGB, either of these patterns carries great localizing value and can thus be extremely helpful clinically, as illustrated in the above case. This is another example in which the clinical findings are the key to interpreting the radiographic study. Without the information from the visual field, the responsible lesion is lost in the background noise of scattered small vessel disease.

Diagnosis: Lateral geniculate body stroke

Tip: The exquisite localizing value of this particular visual field pattern enables the clinician to dis-

tinguish the causative lesion from other, clinically insignificant, areas of ischemic white matter disease.

FURTHER READING

Painful ophthalmoplegia

International Headache Society, The international classification of headache disorders ICHD-II. *Cephalalgia*, **24** Suppl. 1 (2004), 131.

L. B. Kline, W. F. Hoyt, The Tolosa-Hunt syndrome. *J Neurol Neurosurg Psychiatry*, **71** (2001), 577–82.

D. M. Yousem, S. W. Atlas, R. Grossman *et al.*, MR imaging of Tolosa-Hunt syndrome. *AJNR*, **10** (1990), 1181–4.

Orbital apex syndrome

A. Ettl, K. Zwrtek, A. Daxer, E. Salomonowitz, Anatomy of the orbital apex and cavernous sinus on high-resolution magnetic resonance images. *Surv Ophthalmol*, **44** (2000), 303–23.

E. B. Ing, V. Purvin, Progressive visual loss and motility deficit. *Surv Ophthalmol*, **41** (1997), 488–92.

Third nerve misdirection

N. J. Schatz, P. J. Savino, J. J. Corbett, Primary aberrant oculomotor regeneration. *Arch Neurol*, **34** (1977), 29–32.

P. A. Sibony, C. Evinger, S. Lessell, Retrograde horseradish peroxidase transport after oculomotor nerve injury. *Invest Ophthalmol Vis Sci*, **27** (1986), 975–80.

P. A. Sibony, S. Lessell, J. W. Gittinger, Acquired oculomotor synkinesis. *Surv Ophthalmol*, **28** (1984), 382–90.

Lateral geniculate body

L. Frisen, Quadruple sectoranopia and sectoral optic atrophy: a syndrome of the distal anterior choroidal artery. *J Neurol Neurosurg Psychiatry*, **42** (1979), 590–4.

L. Frisen, L. Holmegaard, M. Rosencrantz, Sectorial optic atrophy and homonymous, horizontal sectoranopia: a lateral choroidal artery syndrome? *J Neurol Neurosurg Psychiatry*, **41** (1978), 374–80.

J. C. Horton, K. Landau, P. Maeder, W. F. Hoyt, Magnetic resonance imaging of the human lateral geniculate body. *Arch Neurol*, **47** (1990), 1201–6.

7

Clinical findings that are subtle

The process of arriving at a diagnosis involves the collection of many kinds of information. Data from the history, the examination and, in some cases, ancillary investigations, are consolidated into a diagnostic judgement. In many instances, all of this information contributes to the determination of the correct diagnosis, but occasionally the solution to a challenging or puzzling case rests on a small finding. Despite their clinical importance, such subtle abnormalities may be easily overlooked. Cases that highlight some of these abnormalities should encourage us to hone our powers of observation.

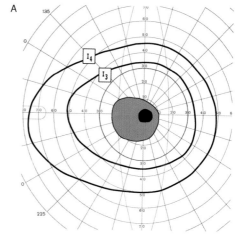

Painless central gray spot in a teenager

Case: A 17-year-old student developed a painless "grayish spot" in the central vision of his left eye. Over the next few days the spot progressed to look like a "backward black C" and then remained stable. He had been otherwise in good health. Examination 10 days after onset showed visual acuity of 20/20 OD and 20/200 OS, with moderate dyschromatopsia and a large central scotoma in the left eye (Figure 7.1A). Pupils constricted briskly to light with a small left RAPD. Fundus examination revealed a normal right optic disc and moderate swelling of the left disc (Figure 7.1B). He was thought to have optic neuritis, prompting an MR scan of brain and orbits that was normal.

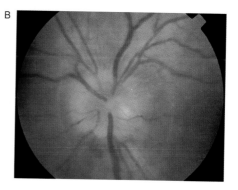

Figure 7.1 Visual findings in a 17-year-old student with acute monocular visual loss. (A) Goldmann perimetry in the left eye shows a large central scotoma. (B) The left optic disc is diffusely swollen and the retinal veins mildly venous distended.

A   B

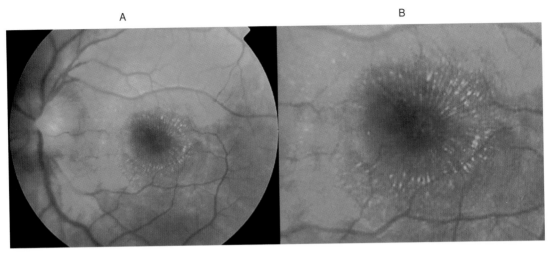

Figure 7.2 (A) Closer inspection of the same patient's left fundus shows a subtle macular star figure in addition to disc edema. (B) A magnified view better demonstrates the hard exudates in a spoke-like pattern centered on the macula.

What clinical features suggest a diagnosis other than idiopathic (demyelinating) optic neuritis in this patient?

Absence of eye pain is unusual in optic neuritis. In addition, there is extensive central visual loss in the involved eye but only a small RAPD. This discrepancy between the visual loss (severe) and RAPD (mild) suggests that, although the optic disc is swollen, the visual loss is due, at least in part, to retinal rather than optic nerve dysfunction. Closer inspection of the left fundus revealed very fine, spoke-like exudates centering around the macula (Figure 7.2). The presence of this subtle macular star indicates a diagnosis of *neuroretinitis* rather than optic neuritis. There is also a serous detachment involving the macula which is more difficult to appreciate than the star, accounting for the central scotoma.

What is the most likely cause of this patient's neuroretinitis, and how would you test for it?

The most common cause of neuroretinitis is *cat scratch disease*, and the diagnosis is established by serologic testing for antibodies to the infectious organism. The patient owned a young cat who

scratched him often. The *Bartonella henselae* IgG titer was elevated at 1:512 (normal <1:64) and IgM titer mildly elevated at 1:16 (normal <1:16), consistent with a recent infection. The patient was treated with a 10 day course of ciprofloxacin for cat-scratch neuroretinitis. At follow-up six months later, vision in his left eye had markedly improved to 20/30 with just a small shallow central scotoma.

Discussion: Initially designated as "stellate maculopathy", it was subsequently recognized that the macular exudates that define this condition represent leakage of protein and lipid, not from the macula, but from inflamed disc capillaries. This fluid then spreads into the peri-papillary subretinal space and outer plexiform layer, where resorption of the serous component leaves lipid exudates that are subsequently ingested by macrophages. The star pattern of exudates reflects the loose, radial configuration of the outer plexiform layer in the macula.

Neuroretinitis usually affects children and young adults, but the age range is broad. Males and females are affected equally. Neuroretinitis has been reported in association with a variety of infectious agents, the most common of which is cat

Table 7.1 Etiologies of neuroretinitis

Bartonella species (mostly *B. henselae*)

Spirochetes
   syphilis (secondary or tertiary)
   Lyme disease (Stage II)
   leptospirosis

Viral or post-viral
   mumps
   chicken pox
   herpes simplex
   herpes zoster
   HIV
   hepatitis B
   Coxsackie B
   influenza A
   Epstein Barr virus
   Cytomegalovirus

Tuberculosis

Toxoplasmosis

Nematodes
   Toxocara canis
   diffuse unilateral subacute neuroretinitis (DUSN)

Histoplasmosis capsulatum

Rocky mountain spotted fever

Salmonella

Post-vaccination
   rabies

Non-infectious uveitis
   sarcoidosis
   inflammatory bowel disease
   periarteritis nodosa

Uncertain mechanism
   Parry–Romberg syndrome (progressive facial
     hemiatrophy)
   idiopathic retinal vasculitis and aneurysms (IRVAN
     syndrome)
   tubulointerstitial nephritis and uveitis (TINU syndrome)

scratch disease (see Table 7.1). Cases in which no infectious etiology is identified are designated as idiopathic neuroretinitis. Regardless of etiology, approximately 50 % of all affected individuals experience an antecedent flu-like illness. In patients with cat-scratch neuroretinitis these prodromal symptoms usually include sore throat, headache, myal-

gias and lymphadenopathy. Visual loss typically takes the form of unilateral blurring of central vision, which is usually painless but occasionally accompanied by a mild ache that is not exacerbated by eye movement.

Visual acuity is reduced during the acute phase, and visual field testing usually shows a central or ceco-central scotoma that corresponds to the serous retinal detachment. To the extent that visual loss in this condition is related to retinal rather than optic nerve dysfunction, the magnitude and constancy of an RAPD in neuroretinitis is less than in optic neuritis, making this a useful differential feature. In some cases there is also a degree of optic nerve dysfunction and in these cases the RAPD is more substantial.

The fundus appearance of neuroretinitis depends, in large part, on the timing of the examination. The earliest finding is disc edema that may be diffuse or segmental and is sometimes accompanied by peri-papillary nerve fiber layer hemorrhages. The disc edema in this condition is typically associated with peri-papillary serous retinal detachment extending to the macula. In addition to the characteristic changes involving the disc and macula, small yellow-white chorioretinal spots are sometimes identified. Over time, usually 9 to 12 days after onset, the serous portion of the exudation is absorbed, leaving the lipid portion which then emerges as the characteristic macular star figure (Figure 7.3). The star is initially sharply defined and spoke-like; over time the exudate develops a more globby appearance and eventually, after a number of months, disappears completely, often leaving residual subfoveal RPE defects in the macula that remain as a helpful clue to the nature of the original episode. The disc may eventually return to normal or may show pallor and gliotic changes.

Most patients with neuroretinitis enjoy excellent recovery of vision without intervention, and a repeat event either in the previously affected or the fellow eye is unusual. Patients in whom cat scratch disease is identified or suspected are often treated with antibiotics, as in the above case, but there is

A   B

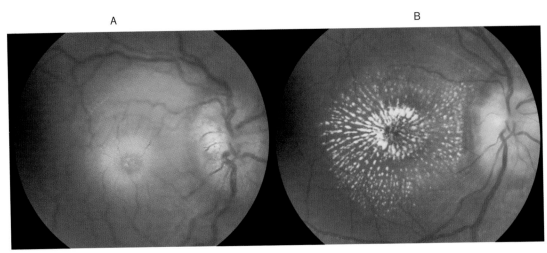

Figure 7.3 Fundus findings in a different patient with acute neuroretinitis OD. (A) One week after onset of visual loss there is prominent disc edema and subtle whitening of the macula. (B) Two weeks later, disc edema has diminished and the serous component of the exudation has resorbed, leaving lipid exudates in a dramatic star configuration centered on the macula.

no evidence that such treatment improves the natural history of the condition. There appears to be a small subset of patients, however, with a somewhat different clinical picture in whom the prognosis is more guarded. These patients experience repeated attacks with residual visual loss each time which causes substantial cumulative damage. This variant, termed *idiopathic recurrent neuroretinitis*, may be suspected during the initial episode by virtue of a large relative afferent pupillary defect, disc-related field loss and poor visual recovery. Such patients should be considered to be at risk for a future similar event and should be counseled accordingly. In patients who have experienced recurrent episodes, prophylactic immunosuppressive treatment may be considered.

The diagnosis of neuroretinitis is a clinical one, based on the presence of a macular star figure in conjunction with other typical clinical features. It is important to keep in mind that other conditions can be associated with a macular star, namely malignant hypertension, increased intracranial pressure (papilledema), ischemic optic neuropathy and diabetic papillopathy. In distinguishing among these

mechanisms, it is helpful to note whether the condition affects one or both eyes. Bilateral simultaneous neuroretinitis is unusual, whereas the fundus changes in malignant hypertension and increased intracranial pressure are typically bilateral and relatively symmetric (see Chapter 1, Headache and bilateral disc edema).

It is important to distinguish patients with neuroretinitis from those with optic neuritis because of the very different neurologic prognosis in the two conditions. Patients who experience an attack of optic neuritis are at increased risk for the future development of MS (see Chapter 12, Prednisone for demyelinating optic neuritis), whereas those with neuroretinitis are not. This difference in prognosis is presumably related to differences in pathophysiology in these two conditions. In demyelinating optic neuritis the target tissue of the inflammatory response is the myelin sheath, whereas in neuroretinitis the target is the optic disc vasculature. When the patient is seen after the development of the macular star, diagnosis and prognosis should be straightforward. In the acute stage, the lack of pain and absent or small RAPD relative to the degree of visual loss should suggest the possibility of neuro-retinitis or other macular disturbance. The age of the patient may also be helpful, in that childhood optic neuritis is uncommon. When neuroretinitis is suspected, a repeat evaluation including dilated fundus examination one to two weeks later can confirm the diagnosis.

Diagnosis: Neuroretinitis due to cat scratch disease

Tip: A fully developed macular star is readily recognized; in the very early and very late stages the fundus findings are more subtle. The presence of a macular star at any stage is inconsistent with a diagnosis of demyelinating optic neuritis.

Chronic "pink eye"

Case: This 75-year-old, active grandmother noticed mild redness of her right eye (Figure 7.4). Thinking she had caught an eye infection from one of her grandchildren (who had been treated for conjunctivitis several weeks previously) she did not seek medical advice immediately. The redness did not improve over the next three months, so she consulted her eye doctor who found normal visual function, ocular motility and fundus appearance. Warm compresses and observational management were recommended.

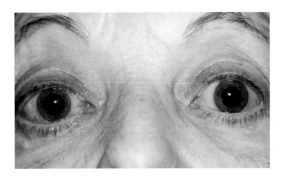

Figure 7.4 External appearance of a 75-year-old, active grandmother with mild conjunctival injection of the right eye.

Her red eye persisted and over the next month she developed new right periorbital pain and intermittent horizontal diplopia. A second examination revealed no objective abnormalities and she was given a mild analgesic for her headache and a return appointment in four months.

This patient had an additional non-ocular symptom which she did not volunteer because she didn't think it was relevant to her eye problem, yet this symptom was an important clue to the correct diagnosis. What question should be asked?

This patient should be questioned about pulsatile tinnitus. Once queried, she admitted to "hearing her heartbeat" on the right side of her head for the past few months, suggesting the presence of a carotid-cavernous sinus fistula as the cause of her red eye. Four months later, examination of the right eye revealed more prominent dilation and tortuosity of conjunctival and episcleral vessels, mild conjunctival edema, 3 mm of right-sided proptosis, and a mild right abduction deficit (Figure 7.5A and B). Intraocular pressure was elevated in the right eye (25 mmHg OD vs. 18 mmHg OS) and funduscopy revealed mild tortuosity of the retinal veins. An orbital CT showed dilation of the right superior ophthalmic vein and mild diffuse enlargement of the extraocular muscles, consistent with orbital venous congestion (Figure 7.5C).

Discussion: A carotid-cavernous sinus fistula represents an abnormal communication between the carotid system and the cavernous sinus, introducing arterial blood into the venous space and thus leading to an increase in venous pressure. A "direct" or "high flow" fistula occurs when the communication is between the internal carotid artery and the cavernous sinus, usually the consequence of trauma. Due to the high-flow shunting of arterial blood, clinical manifestations of a direct fistula are sudden and dramatic. In contrast, a *dural fistula* occurs when the defect involves a meningeal branch of the external or internal carotid artery, resulting in a

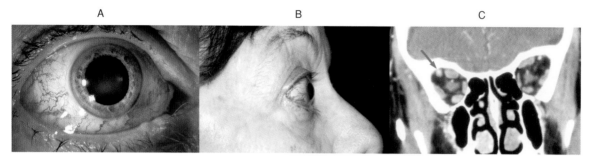

Figure 7.5 Examination and radiographic findings in the same patient four months later. (A) There is arterialization of conjunctival vessels and (B) proptosis of the right eye. (C) Coronal post-contrast CT of the mid-orbit shows prominence of the superior ophthalmic vein on the right side (arrow). There is also mild enlargement of the extraocular muscles on that side.

low-flow communication with the cavernous sinus. Such low-flow fistulas usually arise spontaneously, typically in postmenopausal women and during pregnancy, and the associated signs and symptoms are generally milder.

The drainage pattern of the additional blood volume from the cavernous sinus dictates the clinical presentation of a dural fistula. In most cases, the shunted blood flows anteriorly through the superior and inferior ophthalmic veins, causing a variety of signs and symptoms related to orbital venous congestion. Occasionally, drainage is directed posteriorly through the superior or inferior petrosal sinuses. In these cases, an isolated cranial nerve palsy (usually sixth nerve, occasionally fourth) may be the only clinical manifestation. Due to the absence of orbital congestion, such cases are sometimes referred to as a "white-eyed shunt" and pose more of a diagnostic challenge. Uncommonly, signs and symptoms are bilateral or even contralateral to a unilateral fistula due to prominent intercavernous venous connections. Regardless of the direction of drainage, most patients have some degree of ipsilateral pain, although the severity is quite variable. While helpful when present, a bruit (subjective or objective) is reported in only 25% of cases.

Examination typically shows signs of orbital congestion including proptosis, chemosis, lid edema and conjunctival injection. Abnormal ocular motor motility may be due to cranial nerve palsy secondary to pressure and/or ischemia within the cavernous sinus or to extraocular muscle dysfunction caused by muscle swelling. Increased orbital venous pressure, also causes an increase in episcleral venous pressure, resulting in elevated intraocular pressure and congestion of surface vessels. In its full-fledged form, the episcleral vessels are dilated and tortuous with a classic "corkscrew" appearance characterized by looping in a radial pattern from the corneal limbus, an appearance that is virtually diagnostic (Figure 7.6). Milder forms may be more difficult to distinguish from anterior segment inflammatory conditions (conjunctivitis, episcleritis and scleritis). Posterior segment changes of venous congestion include retinal venous stasis or obstruction, choroidal folds and effusion and disc swelling. Visual loss, when it occurs, is multifactorial, with elements of glaucomatous damage to the disc, compression of the intracranial optic nerve by a dilated cavernous sinus and ischemia of the optic nerve and/or retina.

In most cases, orbital signs are prominent and thus the main differential diagnoses are thyroid orbitopathy, orbital inflammatory disease (cellulitis or pseudotumor) and cavernous sinus thrombosis. There is some overlap in the radiographic appearance in these conditions and thus a diagnosis cannot be made solely on the basis of scan findings. MRI and CT do not directly demonstrate a dural

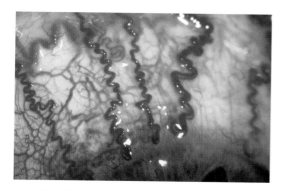

Figure 7.6 Close-up view of the superior conjunctiva in a different patient with a dural-cavernous fistula, showing characteristic "corkscrew vessels".

fistula but instead reveal signs related to increased orbital venous drainage, providing indirect radiographic support for the diagnosis. Enlargement of the extraocular muscles is common and may be mistakenly attributed to Graves' disease. Associated enlargement of the superior ophthalmic vein is an extremely helpful finding, typically present in fistulas but not in thyroid eye disease. This same radiographic appearance, however, may also be seen in cavernous sinus thrombosis. In some cases, careful inspection will show relative fullness of the cavernous sinus on the side of the fistula and an MRA may show subtle hypervascularity (Figure 7.7). Catheter angiography is the only way to conclusively demonstrate a dural- or carotid-cavernous fistula,

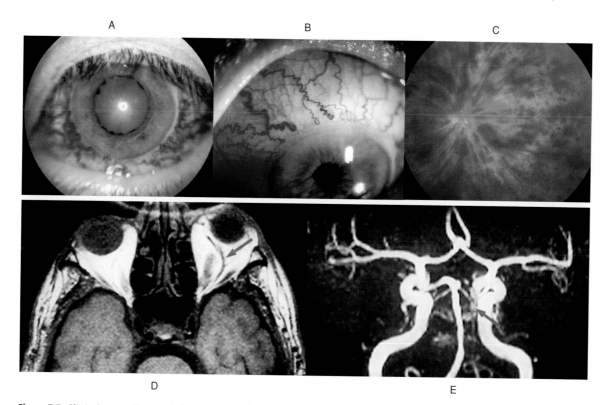

Figure 7.7 Clinical and radiographic findings in a different patient, a 75-year-old man with a left dural-cavernous fistula. (A) There is marked arterialization of episcleral veins. (The pupil is pharmacologically dilated.) (B) Close-up view shows the typical radial pattern of the corkscrew vessels. (C) Ophthalmoscopy of the left eye reveals disc edema and widespread retinal hemorrhages secondary to central retinal vein occlusion. (D) An enlarged superior ophthalmic vein is visible on the axial non-contrast T1-weighted MR image (arrow). (E) MRA shows abnormal left cavernous sinus opacification (arrow).

and is also necessary for determining the pattern of venous drainage in patients for whom treatment is anticipated. Angiography is also necessary to identify those patients with collateral cortical venous drainage, which carries a risk of subarachnoid hemorrhage. Such collateral circulation is uncommon, however, and angiography carries some attendant risk, particularly in older patients with vascular disease. Thus, the risk of the test must be weighed against the risks of the fistula itself and management decisions must be individualized.

Not all fistulas require treatment. The usual indications for treatment are: intractable pain, progressive visual loss, uncontrollable glaucoma, unsightly proptosis, exposure keratopathy, severe ophthalmoplegia and collateral cortical venous drainage. Moreover, approximately 20 to 50% of fistulas undergo closure, either spontaneously or following angiography, and so temporizing in some cases is appropriate. Occasionally, abrupt and dramatic worsening of clinical manifestations occurs due to acute thrombosis of the superior ophthalmic vein or cavernous sinus, followed by resolution of clinical findings over several weeks as the thrombosis closes the shunt.

Diagnosis: Dural-cavernous fistula

Tip: A chronic red eye that fails to respond to treatment for inflammation should raise suspicion of a dural carotid-cavernous sinus fistula. Patients should be specifically questioned about pulsatile tinnitus.

Bouncing vision

Case: A 40-year-old attorney experienced intermittent blurring of vision while playing tennis. She was generally healthy and a complete ophthalmic examination was unremarkable. Six months later she also developed difficulty reading, specifically noting that it was hard to keep her eyes steady on the page. She also developed new posterior headaches and intermittent horizontal diplopia, particularly when driving home at night. On closer questioning, she described intermittent "bouncing" of her vision.

What is her symptom of "bouncing vision" called and what physical finding would you look for on examination?

Illusory movement of the environment is termed *oscillopsia* and it is most commonly due to rhythmic to-and-fro movements of the eyes, termed *nystagmus*.

This patient's eye examination, however, was normal, specifically nystagmus was not observed. Why not?

Nystagmus varies in terms of amplitude and frequency and these parameters may vary further with gaze position. When nystagmus is of small amplitude and low frequency it is more difficult to detect, especially if it is subtle or absent in primary position.

What examination techniques can help in the detection of nystagmus when the oscillatory amplitude is particularly small?

Techniques that magnify the eyes can be very helpful in this regard. One simple bedside maneuver is to observe the optic disc with the direct ophthalmoscope. The magnification provided by the ophthalmoscope makes even very small ocular oscillations (micronystagmus) readily apparent. Examination at the slit-lamp, focusing on a conjunctival vessel, can be similarly effective. Illuminated Frenzel glasses (+20 lenses) are useful for abolishing fixation and thus revealing peripheral vestibular nystagmus. One can combine techniques by using a high plus lens to fog (blur) one eye while observing the other eye with the direct ophthalmoscope.

Another useful technique is viewing the eyes in different positions of eccentric gaze. In most patients with jerk-type nystagmus, the amplitude increases when gaze is directed toward the fast-beating component, a characteristic termed

Alexander's law. In some patients, nystagmus is only present in a particular position of gaze, so it is important to observe the stability of fixation with the patient looking in different directions but especially in the *symptomatic* position of gaze. In contrast to gaze-dependent nystagmus, patients with rebound nystagmus show ocular oscillations only upon returning to primary position after sustained eccentric gaze. Finally, because some forms of nystagmus vary over time, it is important to observe the patient for several minutes. Periodic alternating nystagmus is a distinctive form of horizontal jerk nystagmus in which the fast component decreases in amplitude and then changes direction every two to three minutes, with a brief null period between phases.

This patient was re-examined and found to have small amplitude downbeat nystagmus that was visible in primary position only when viewed with the direct ophthalmoscope. Small-amplitude nystagmus was also visible without magnification when she looked down-lateral to either side. An MRI showed downward displacement of the cerebellar tonsils through the foramen magnum, consistent with a Chiari I malformation (Figure 7.8). Following surgical decompression of the craniocervical junction the patient's headaches resolved completely. Oscillopsia improved though did not resolve entirely and she continued to have occasional diplopia.

Discussion: Downbeat nystagmus is a distinctive sign that results from defective vertical gaze holding, causing a slow upward drift of the eyes followed by a corrective downward saccade. Although downbeat nystagmus is usually present with the eyes in primary position, its amplitude may be so small as to go unnoticed on routine examination, as in our patient. In many patients, the amplitude of the nystagmus is greater in downgaze, lateral gaze or gaze down-lateral, as in the above case. It is therefore important to carefully observe fixational stability, not just in primary position, but in different directions of gaze and particularly in the field of gaze in which the patient is symptomatic. For example, patients who describe oscillopsia or other ocular

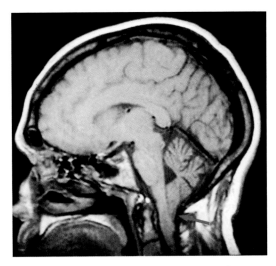

Figure 7.8 Sagittal non-contrast T1-weighted midline MR image of the above patient with downbeat nystagmus shows descent of the cerebellar tonsils (arrow), characteristic of a Chiari I malformation. Note compression of the lower brainstem by the tonsillar herniation.

instability with reading should be closely observed with the eyes in downgaze.

Downbeat nystagmus can be caused by a variety of conditions, including structural abnormalities at the craniocervical junction (see Table 7.2). In cases without a compressive lesion, etiologies include stroke, hereditary cerebellar degeneration, demyelinating disease, paraneoplastic syndromes and certain toxic/metabolic conditions. The time course of the disorder is often helpful in distinguishing among these etiologies. In cerebellar degeneration and Chiari malformations the progression of symptoms is quite slow (over years) compared to stroke and demyelinating disease, in which onset is abrupt. Paraneoplastic syndromes are usually subacute in onset, progressing over weeks to months, and oscillopsia is usually accompanied by more severe symptoms of gait instability, vertigo and nausea.

The Chiari malformations represent a continuum of hindbrain maldevelopments characterized by increasing degrees of herniation of inferior

Table 7.2 Causes of downbeat nystagmus

Idiopathic and familial cerebellar degeneration
Compressive lesions
   Chiari malformation
   foramen magnum meningioma
   vertebrobasilar dolichoectasia
Stroke
Demyelinating disease
Paraneoplastic syndromes
Syringobulbia
Trauma
Hydrocephalus
Metabolic derangements
   magnesium depletion
   thiamine deficiency (Wernicke's)
Toxins
   alcohol
   toluene
Anti-convulsants
   diphenylhydantoin
   carbamazepine
   lamotrigine
Heat stroke
Encephalitis

Table 7.3 Symptoms of Chiari I malformation

Headache or neck pain
Ataxia
Sensory disturbance
Vertigo
Oscillopsia
Diplopia
Syncope
Limb weakness
Palpitations
Tinnitus
Dysphagia
Dysarthria
Apnea

cerebellar structures through the foramen magnum. *Chiari I malformation* is the least severe and is limited to downward displacement of the cerebellar tonsils. Minor degrees of displacement are often asymptomatic. In patients who undergo MR scanning for vague, non-specific symptoms, the radiographic presence of a Chiari I malformation does not necessarily imply a causal relationship to the patient's symptom(s). Deciding whether or not a Chiari I malformation is symptomatic can, at times, be challenging. Focal deficits related to brainstem, cerebellar or spinal cord dysfunction can be confidently attributed to the malformation. In patients with non-localizing symptoms such as fatigue and chronic headache, a causal relationship may be more difficult to establish.

Patients with a symptomatic Chiari I malformation usually present in late adolescence to early adulthood. Cases in childhood are increasingly recognized, however, and patients who present in mid-life often report that they have "always" had poor balance and coordination. The most common symptom is headache, usually in the occipital or posterior cervical region. Severe paroxysmal pain may be provoked by a Valsalva maneuver such as coughing, sneezing, laughing or straining, sometimes referred to as *cough headache.* Diverse neurologic and systemic symptoms (see Table 7.3) may lead to diagnostic confusion with multiple sclerosis, fibromyalgia, dysautonomia and even hysteria. Exercise, particularly activities involving neck extension, can precipitate symptoms related to hindbrain herniation. Such a history of worsening neurologic symptoms with exercise may be misinterpreted as Uhthoff's phenomenon, as in the patient under discussion, and may further the impression of occult demyelinating disease.

While downbeat nystagmus is the most common neuro-ophthalmic manifestation of Chiari syndrome, a variety of ocular motor abnormalities occur in these patients, including other forms of nystagmus (periodic alternating, rebound, see-saw and convergence), as well as other involuntary ocular oscillations (ocular flutter and dysmetria) (see Table 7.4). Patterns of ocular misalignment include esotropia (due to divergence insufficiency, sixth nerve palsy and convergence spasm), skew deviation and internuclear ophthalmoplegia (see Chapter 5, Low cerebellar tonsils). In patients

Table 7.4 Ocular motor abnormalities associated with Chiari I malformation

Downbeat nystagmus
Horizontal nystagmus (primary or on lateral gaze)
Periodic alternating nystagmus
Rebound nystagmus
Positional nystagmus
Skew deviation (often alternating)
Impaired pursuit
Internuclear ophthalmoplegia
Comitant esotropia

suspected of harboring a Chiari I malformation, the neurologic evaluation should particularly address the presence of cerebellar deficits, lower cranial nerve dysfunction, associated syrinx, skeletal anomalies of the cervical spine, scoliosis and evidence of increased intracranial pressure.

The natural history of a symptomatic Chiari malformation usually involves slow progression over time. Patients with minimal symptoms may be followed conservatively or treated symptomatically. Definitive treatment consists of posterior fossa decompression. Success rates vary, depending on the clinical manifestations and the presence of an associated syrinx. Symptoms that are related to tonsillar impaction and increased intracranial pressure (e.g. headache, neck pain and oscillopsia) tend to respond more favorably to surgery than focal deficits due to brainstem or spinal cord compression. Surgical decompression prevents further progression of neurologic deficits and about half of patients report improvement of symptoms.

Diagnosis: Downbeat nystagmus due to Chiari I malformation

Tip: Small amplitude nystagmus may be visible only on eccentric gaze or with direct ophthalmoscopy. The presence of downbeat nystagmus directs attention to the cerebellum and craniocervical junction.

Farmer with an adduction deficit

Case: A 70-year-old farmer developed acute onset of horizontal diplopia that was worse on left gaze. There was no pain and no other focal neurologic deficits or recent systemic symptoms. Examination showed limitation of adduction in the right eye with otherwise full eye movements. There was no ptosis and pupils were isocoric with brisk responses to light stimulation. He was thought to have a right internuclear ophthalmoplegia (INO), most likely due to a brainstem stroke. An MRI was normal and he was subsequently referred for neuro-ophthalmic consultation.

Ocular motor examination confirmed an adduction deficit of the right eye (Figure 7.9A). Testing of refixation eye movements showed prominent slowing of right medial rectus saccades for large amplitude (20 degree) movements. When the patient was instructed to make small amplitude (5 degree) refixation movements, however, medial rectus saccades

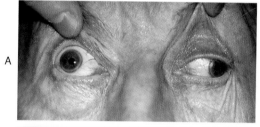

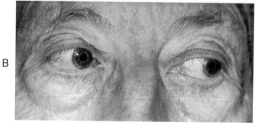

Figure 7.9 Tensilon test in the above 70-year-old man with a "pseudo-INO". (A) There is no adduction past midline in the right eye. (B) Following administration of 6 mg of edrophonium chloride (Tensilon), there is complete reversal of the adduction deficit. In retrospect his previous ptosis, attributed to dermatochalasis, was also myasthenic, now improved with Tensilon.

were brisk. This observation of a discrepancy in the saccadic velocity between large and small amplitude refixation movements, though subtle, was the key to the correct diagnosis in this case, suggesting neuromuscular junction disease. The patient subsequently had a positive Tensilon (edrophonium chloride) test (Figure 7.9B) and elevated acetylcholine receptor antibody titers, confirming a diagnosis of myasthenia gravis. This patient's ocular motor disturbance would therefore be classified as a *"pseudo-INO"*, i.e. myasthenia mimicking a supranuclear abnormality.

Discussion: Electro-oculographic studies have demonstrated that saccadic velocity in myasthenia is not only preserved but is often supra-normal, due to an increased firing rate in the paramedian pontine reticular formation (PPRF) designed to overcome the neuromuscular junction blockade. This observation, however, does not apply to all saccadic movements. During eye movement recordings, small movements made by a myasthenic muscle do demonstrate this preservation or even augmentation of saccadic velocity. During large amplitude movements, however, an affected eye muscle may exhibit a loss of velocity during the course of a single excursion, termed "intra-saccadic fatigue". In some cases, careful bedside examination can detect this change in velocity during the course of an eye movement. The patient is asked to quickly refixate from extreme lateral gaze to a target on the opposite side. In a normal saccade the velocity is rapid and uniform. In the presence of intra-saccadic fatigue, the eye movement appears to have two phases: an initial brisk burst of movement followed by a slower continuation toward the intended target. Another way to demonstrate this phenomenon is to compare velocities of small vs. large amplitude saccades, as described in the case example.

Slowing of medial rectus saccades is the most sensitive and invariable sign of an internuclear ophthalmoplegia (INO), demonstrable even in the absence of an adduction deficit. Such slowing can be demonstrated for both large and small amplitude eye movements. In contrast, in an adduction deficit due to myasthenia, small amplitude medial rectus saccades exhibit a normal or supra-normal velocity. Because myasthenia can affect just one or two muscles, it often resembles a cranial nerve palsy or supranuclear gaze disturbance. The medial rectus muscle is frequently affected in myasthenia and thus the clinical picture of a unilateral or bilateral "pseudo-INO" is not uncommon.

Diagnosis: Myasthenic pseudo-INO

Tip: In a patient with an isolated adduction deficit, the presence of brisk saccadic velocity for small amplitude adduction movements distinguishes a myasthenic "pseudo-INO" from a true INO.

FURTHER READING

Neuroretinitis

V. C. Parmley, J. S. Schiffman, C. G. Maitland *et al.*, Does neuroretinitis rule out multiple sclerosis? *Arch Neurol,* **44** (1987), 1045–8.

V. Purvin, Neuroretinitis. In D. Albert, J. Miller, eds., *Albert and Jakobiec's Principles and Practice of Ophthalmology,* 3rd edn. Philadelphia: Elsevier, 2007, pp. 1859–63.

V. Purvin, G. Chioran, Recurrent neuroretinitis. *Arch Ophthalmol,* **112** (1994), 365–71.

J. B. Reed, D. K. Scales, M. T. Wong *et al., Bartonella henselae* neuroretinitis in cat scratch disease: diagnosis, management and sequelae, *Ophthalmology,* **105** (1998), 459–66.

Dural-cavernous fistula

R. J. W. De Keizer, Carotid-cavernous and orbital arteriovenous fistulas: ocular features, diagnostic and hemodynamic considerations in relation to visual impairment and morbidity. *Orbit,* **22** (2003), 121–42.

E. Eggenberger, A. G. Lee, T. R. Forget Jr., R. Rosenwasser, A brutal headache and double vision. *Surv Ophthalmol,* **45** (2000), 147–53.

M. J. Kupersmith, Carotid cavernous fistulas. In *Neurovascular Neuro-Ophthalmology.* New York: Springer-Verlag, 1993, pp. 69–108.

P. M. Meyers, V. V. Halbach, C. F. Dowd *et al.*, Dural carotid cavernous fistula: definitive endovascular management and long-term follow-up. *Am J Ophthalmol*, **134** (2002), 85–92.

Downbeat nystagmus

J. S. Cheng, J. Nash, G. A. Meyer, Chiari type I malformation revisited: diagnosis and treatment. *Neurologist*, **8** (2002), 357–62.

R. J. Leigh and D. Z. Zee, Diagnosis of Nystagmus. In *The Neurology of Eye Movements*, 4th edn. Contemporary Neurology Series. New York: Oxford University Press, 2006, pp. 475–558.

A. Rowlands, A. Sgouros, B. Williams, Ocular manifestations of hindbrain-related syringomyelia and outcome

following craniovertebral decompression. *Eye*, **14** (2000), 884–8.

R. D. Yee, Downbeat nystagmus: characteristics and localization of lesions. *Trans Am Ophthalmol Soc*, **87** (1990), 984–1032.

Myasthenic "pseudo-INO"

T. B. Crane, R. D. Yee, R. W. Baloh, R. S. Hepler, Analysis of characteristic eye movement abnormalities in internuclear ophthalmoplegia. *Arch Ophthalmol*, **101** (1983), 206–10.

J. S. Glaser, Myasthenic pseudo-internuclear ophthalmoplegia, *Arch Ophthalmol*, **75** (1066), 363–6.

R. D. Yee, S. M. Whitcup, I. M. Williams, R. W. Baloh, V. Honrubia, Saccadic eye movements in myasthenia gravis. *Ophthalmology*, **94** (1987), 219–25.

8

Misinterpretation of visual fields

The diagnostic approach to the patient with unexplained visual loss is to first determine the location of the lesion and then the nature of the disease process. In the process of localization, familiarity with the afferent visual pathways is crucial. Specific patterns of visual loss are associated with damage at various levels of the visual system. Anterior to the optic chiasm, visual deficits are monocular. Lesions at the optic disc typically produce visual field defects that emerge from the blindspot and often respect the horizontal meridian. Such "disc-related defects" consist of central or cecocentral scotomas (indicating a lesion of the papillomacular bundle), arcuate defects (damage to superior or inferior arcuate fibers) and radial bundle defects (extending from the blindspot to the periphery temporally). In contrast, more posteriorly along the optic nerve, visual defects tend to point to fixation and respect the vertical meridian. Because 90% of the fibers that comprise the optic nerve subserve central vision, damage to the nerve at any location often produces a defect involving this area of vision. Thus the presence of a central scotoma helps localize to the optic nerve but does not have much localizing power beyond that. Lesions at the chiasm produce bitemporal defects or a junctional scotoma. Lesions posterior to the chiasm result in homonymous defects, i.e. involving the same hemifield in each eye. The one exception to the last statement is the "monocular crescent", a defect in the temporal periphery of the eye contralateral to a lesion of the anterior-most occipital lobe.

Formal perimetry provides a means to describe and quantify the visual field in a reproducible manner. Its localizing power derives from the exquisite topographic representation of the visual pathways. As with all psychophysical tests, however, there is a subjective element that is open to human error both on the part of the patient and the clinician. The cases in this chapter are intended to highlight some potentially confusing visual field defects.

Abnormal field and night blindness

Case: A 28-year-old carpenter suffered a broken wrist after falling off a ladder at work. Unable to return to carpentry until his wrist healed, he was assigned to work as the nightwatchman. In this new work setting, he had difficulty reading signs and seeing objects in the dim evening lighting and felt uncomfortable driving at night due to excessive glare from the headlights of oncoming cars. He requested temporary disability from work and was sent for a medical evaluation.

The patient was healthy and took no medications. Acuity was 20/25 in each eye at distance and near. An Octopus G1 automated test was interpreted as showing "constricted visual fields" in both eyes (Figure 8.1). Biomicroscopy and fundus examination were reportedly normal in both eyes.

The patient had no trouble when asked to count fingers presented in his peripheral visual field at a distance of one meter, and glanced in the appropriate direction whenever a small target was presented briefly in the far periphery. In addition, he

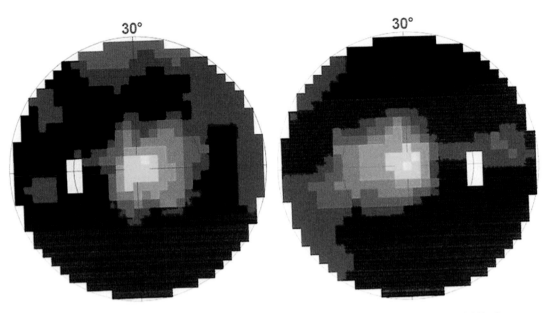

Figure 8.1 Central 30 degree Octopus G1 automated visual field in the above 28-year-old man with visual difficulty at night. There is diffuse loss of sensitivity in both eyes, most severe in the periphery, with relative central sparing.

maneuvered about the office without difficulty, easily noticing objects in his path. Based on the inconsistency between the apparent severity of his visual field defect and his relative ease in performing visually guided activities, functional visual loss was suspected. He was reassured that his vision would improve with time, but six months later he reported no such improvement. His Octopus visual fields were unchanged and this time a Goldmann visual field was obtained (Figure 8.2).

How would you describe this patient's visual field defect? What diagnoses should be considered?

Goldmann perimetry reveals that this patient has dense bilateral ring scotomas as well as diffuse loss of sensitivity. A *ring scotoma* is a doughnut-shaped or annular defect surrounding fixation. It may be partial (as in this patient's left eye) or complete, and indicates photoreceptor dysfunction. Specific etiologies that should be considered in a patient with ring scotomas include: hereditary retinal dystro-

phies, paraneoplastic retinopathy, vitamin A deficiency, certain toxic states and idiopathic inflammation of the outer retina (AZOOR) (see Chapter 1, Twinkling scotoma). Further inquiry revealed that he had noticed poor night vision for several years but had not been sufficiently bothered by it to seek medical attention. There was no family history of visual loss. A full-field ERG with dark adaptometry revealed absent rod function and severe depression of cone function, consistent with a disorder of photoreceptors. Fundus examination was repeated and this time a zone of retinal and pigment epithelial atrophy in the mid-periphery with scattered, small clumps of pigment was appreciated in both eyes (Figure 8.3). A diagnosis of retinitis pigmentosa was made and the patient was appropriately counseled. He eventually transferred to the computer programming department of his company.

Discussion: A ring scotoma in the setting of night blindness and photophobia is the typical presentation of *retinitis pigmentosa*. This is a heterogeneous group of inherited retinopathies that diffusely

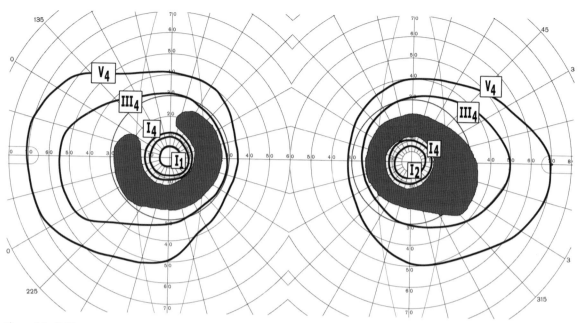

Figure 8.2 Goldmann perimetry in the same patient shows a dense ring scotoma in each eye. There is also diffuse loss of sensitivity, manifest as generalized constriction of all isopters. The peripheral limit of his visual field, however, is relatively normal.

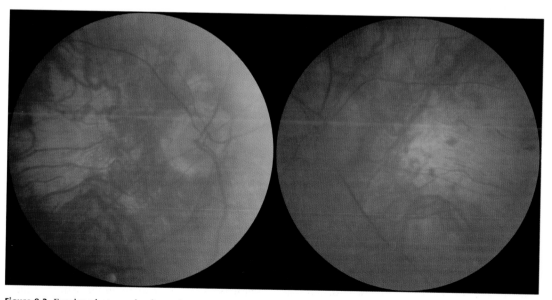

Figure 8.3 Fundus photographs show a large zone of atrophic retina and retinal pigment epithelium in the mid-periphery of each eye, with a few pigment clumps.

and progressively affect the photoreceptors and pigment epithelium. The disorder can be inherited in autosomal dominant, autosomal recessive or X-linked pattern. This patient had no known family history of visual loss but he was an only child whose mother died at an early age in a car accident, and so the genetic information was incomplete. Onset of symptoms in retinitis pigmentosa is highly variable, ranging from early childhood to mid-life. Early symptoms usually consist of prolonged dark adaptation and night blindness. Visual field loss typically begins in the mid-periphery, corresponding to the retinal area of maximal rod density, and progresses relentlessly with continued loss of photoreceptors. The peripheral isopters slowly contract and eventually merge into the scotoma, leaving only a tiny central island of vision at fixation. For most of the course of the disease, Goldmann perimetry is the preferred technique for monitoring visual loss. In end-stage disease, strategies designed to test the macular region using automated perimetry become more useful for assessing the remaining vision. Total blindness is uncommon, but patients with severe loss of peripheral field are functionally disabled.

A full-field electroretinogram, in conjunction with Goldmann kinetic perimetry, is both diagnostic and prognostic. There is marked and often complete loss of both rod and cone signals, usually worse for rods. The fundus typically shows arteriolar narrowing, a waxy pale color of the optic disc and characteristic bone-spicule pigment deposits in the mid-to-far peripheral retina. Early in the course of disease, these pigment deposits may be subtle or even absent. Cystoid macular edema is sometimes present. While characteristic, none of the fundus, ERG or visual field findings is pathognomonic for retinitis pigmentosa. Acquired causes of panretinal dysfunction and degeneration should be ruled out, particularly paraneoplastic retinopathy (CAR syndrome), syphilis, other forms of uveitis and drug toxicity. Systemic diseases that may be associated with retinopathy should be considered in individual cases depending on the clinical findings.

Standardized automated perimetry (including the Humphrey 30–2 or 24–2, Humphrey Fastpac,

Humphrey SITA and Octopus G1) is a differential light threshold test designed to examine the central 24–30 degrees of the visual field. Limiting the test to the central field in this manner saves time and is generally effective because most neurologic visual loss involves this area of the field. While this test strategy is usually accurate in detecting disease involving the afferent visual pathways, there are cases in which important information is omitted, as in the case under discussion. This patient's automated visual fields were mistakenly interpreted as showing severe generalized constriction, whereas, in reality, the far periphery had not been measured and no information about his visual field outside the central 24 degrees can be inferred. In this case, the presence of intact peripheral field, not picked up by the automated test, created the impression of inconsistency between the patient's visual behavior and the results of visual function tests, thus leading to a mistaken diagnosis of non-organic visual loss.

Diagnosis: Retinitis pigmentosa

Tip: Commonly used automated visual field strategies do not test the peripheral field. Awareness of this limitation is important for the proper interpretation of the results in selected cases.

Constricted fields after herniation

Case: A 50-year-old clerk experienced increasing headaches for one month, culminating in a particularly severe episode during which she became unresponsive. She was taken to a local emergency room where she was noted to have a dilated right pupil and extensor posturing. Hydrocephalus was found and a ventriculoperitoneal shunt was placed. After regaining consciousness post-operatively, her general neurologic examination returned to normal but she complained of difficulty seeing. Ophthalmic examination initially suggested severe visual loss because she was unable to read even the big "E" on the Snellen chart. On closer investigation it was discovered that, despite her inability to see large letters, she could read the letters on the 20/25 line

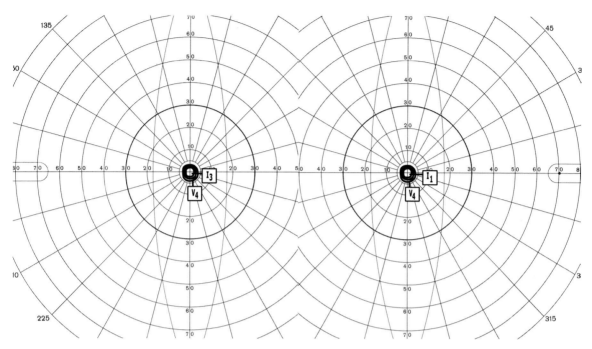

Figure 8.4 Decreased vision following ventriculoperitoneal shunt placement for acute hydrocephalus. Goldmann perimetry shows severe constriction of the visual field to less than five degrees surrounding fixation in each eye. The boundaries of the field are steeply margined, i.e. the isopters are the same size regardless of the intensity of the stimulus.

as well as the numbers on her mobile telephone. Pupillary responses and fundus examination were normal. Confrontation testing showed severe visual field constriction and Goldmann perimetry similarly showed only three degrees of remaining central field in each eye (Figure 8.4). Based on her visual field defect and the apparent inconsistency in results of vision testing, non-organic visual loss was suspected.

What bedside test can help distinguish non-organic field loss from true constriction of the visual field?

Testing the visual field at different distances from the patient is usually diagnostic. Most patients with non-organic field loss exhibit a similar degree of constriction at all distances, referred to as a "tunnel" or "gun-barrel" field. In contrast, the field in

patients with organic constriction shows expansion with increasing distances. This distinctive feature can be demonstrated using simple confrontation techniques at one meter and six meters. A tangent screen, if available, provides comparable information.

The most common causes of severe organic visual field constriction are end-stage glaucoma, severe retinitis pigmentosa and marked post-papilledema optic atrophy, and in these disorders corroborative clinical and fundus findings usually reveal the correct diagnosis. In contrast, cortical visual loss, a less common cause of severe field constriction, may not be accompanied by other ophthalmic or neurologic abnormalities and is therefore more easily mistaken for non-organic visual loss. This patient's confrontational visual field testing at two distances showed physiologic expansion of the field with increasing distance, consistent with organic

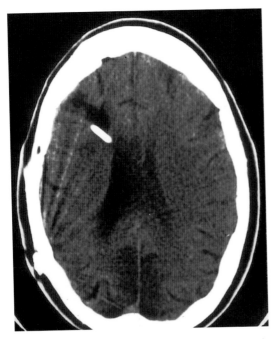

Figure 8.5 Axial non-contrast CT of the above patient with severe visual field constriction. There is a ventriculo-peritoneal shunt in the anterior horn of the right lateral ventricle. The area of low density in the distribution of the posterior cerebral arteries is consistent with bilateral occipital stroke.

disease. A subsequent CT scan showed bilateral occipital infarction with sparing of the occipital tip (Figure 8.5).

Discussion: This patient suffered bilateral occipital lobe infarction due to compression of the posterior cerebral arteries as a consequence of uncal herniation. Due to the dual blood supply to the occipital tip, there was macular sparing, which is represented in the very small area (less than five degree) of preserved central vision. This visual field pattern strongly resembles what is often seen in non-organic field constriction, including the tendency for all the Goldmann isopters to line up together, an unusual characteristic for most neurologic visual loss.

In most cases, a comparison of the visual field at different distances from the patient will successfully distinguish organic from non-organic constriction. Patients with genuine loss show expansion of the field at increasing distance whereas those with non-organic constriction do not. One note of caution should be observed when using this technique, however. In some cases of genuine and profound visual field loss, the constriction is so severe that it is difficult to appreciate this expansion. An additional technique that may be helpful for determining the nature of severe field constriction is to test the peripheral field without the patient's awareness of the purpose of the test. For example, one can perform the standard finger–nose test that is used to assess cerebellar function, presenting the examiner's finger in various parts of the peripheral field, asking the patient to touch the target each time. Most patients with non-organic constriction will readily find and accurately point to the target finger in areas that just a few minutes earlier were apparently blind, whereas those with organic visual loss will either fail to respond at all or will use some form of searching strategy to locate the target.

Diagnosis: Bilateral occipital stroke with macular sparing

Tip: A comparison of the visual field at varying distances from the patient usually distinguishes organic from non-organic constriction.

Sudden difficulty reading the paper

Case: This 55-year-old businessman awoke with a mild headache and at breakfast that morning noted difficulty reading the newspaper. Specifically, he reported a temporal blur in his right eye that blocked parts of words and caused him to lose his place on the line. He was taking no medications and had no known health problems. On examination, visual acuity was 20/20 at distance and at near. Results of pupillary, ocular motility, slit-lamp and funduscopic examinations were unremarkable. An Octopus G1 visual field examination was performed

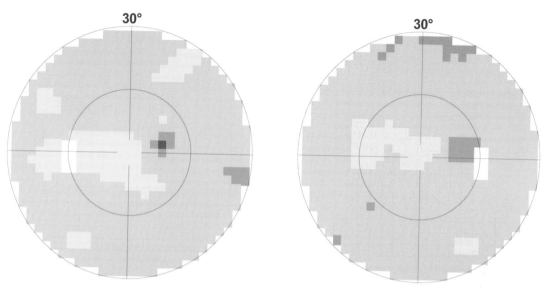

Figure 8.6 Central 30 degree Octopus G1 visual field of a healthy man with acute difficulty reading shows a depressed point (red and green spot) in the nasal hemifield of the left eye.

and interpreted as showing a single focus of depression in the nasal hemifield of his left eye (Figure 8.6). It was hard to reconcile this patient's visual symptoms with his relatively normal examination findings and he was discharged without a specific diagnosis. He returned one week later reporting persistent difficulty reading.

What simple "bedside" test could be performed to further investigate this patient's symptom?

The *Amsler grid* is a useful test for investigating abnormalities of the central visual field. In this patient, an Amsler grid test revealed a scotoma just to the right of fixation in *each* eye. A central 10 degree visual field confirmed a right homonymous hemianopic central scotoma (Figure 8.7A and B).

A non-contrasted MR scan was obtained, which showed a small area of hyperintensity at the left occipital pole consistent with acute hemorrhagic infarction. Further investigation for the origin of his presumed embolic stroke revealed a patent foramen ovale which was subsequently repaired. The patient reported progressive improvement of vision over the next two months and his visual field one year later was nearly normal (Figure 8.8).

Discussion: A unilateral lesion at the tip of the occipital lobe causes a congruous, central, homonymous hemianopic scotoma. Because the lesion is confined to one hemisphere, visual acuity is always preserved. Because the area of damage manifests clinically as a small hemianopic scotoma near fixation, it is often undetectable with confrontational visual field testing and may also be overlooked on standard perimetry. Because the lesion is postgeniculate, the pupils and fundus appearance are normal. In the case of a stroke, visual loss is sudden, painless and typically unassociated with other focal neurologic deficits. Thus, despite the patient's report of an acute visual disturbance, the examination may be surprisingly normal. Further compounding these difficulties in diagnosis, some of these occipital lesions are so small that they go undetected on neuro-imaging studies.

The history in cases of a unilateral occipital tip lesion can be very helpful in pointing to the correct localization. Because the hemianopic scotoma

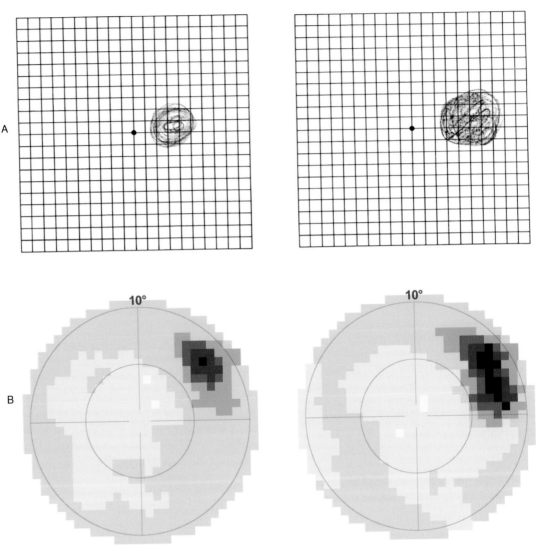

Figure 8.7 Macular visual field testing of the above patient. (A) On the Amsler grid the patient has indicated the location of his visual blur, an area to the right of fixation in each eye. (B) Central 10 degree automated threshold test (Octopus 101, M2 macular testing) of the same patient confirms a small right homonymous hemianopic scotoma, corroborating the Amsler grid findings.

is contained within the central 10 degrees, the visual disturbance is most noticeable when fine visual discrimination is required, such as reading. Some patients recognize that their visual disturbance is related to seeing only half of words. Other patients simply describe their vision as "blurred" when read-

ing and yet others, like this patient above, interpret their homonymous visual loss as being monocular (in the eye with the temporal scotoma). The visual defect is less bothersome or even inapparent during tasks such as driving or watching television because, when viewing large objects at distance, the

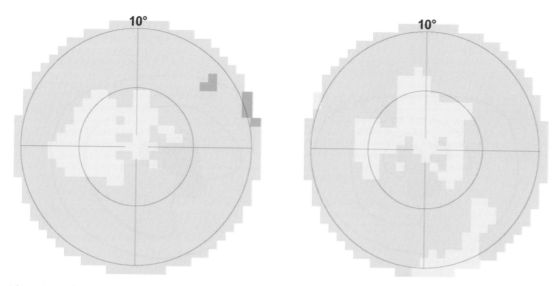

Figure 8.8 Follow-up macular visual field testing (central 10 degrees) one year later shows near-complete resolution of this patient's previous homonymous defect.

missing information in the scotoma is compensated by information obtained from the rest of the visual field.

Due to the very small size and central location of the homonymous scotoma, it can be overlooked on standard automated threshold tests, dismissed as a non-specific parafoveal depression or misinterpreted as a test artifact from unstable fixation. Amsler grid testing is particularly useful in detecting such subtle visual field defects, provided that visual acuity is around 20/40 or better. The most commonly used Amsler grid consists of a series of parallel black lines on a white background, forming a grid of 400 squares covering a 10 cm × 10 cm area. When the patient views the fixation dot in the center of the grid with one eye at a distance of 30 cm, each square represents 1 degree of visual angle and the test assesses the central 10 degrees of the visual field. The patient is asked to fixate on the center of the grid and mark with a pencil any regions where the lines are blurred, missing, or distorted. In this way, the patient can map out his/her own paracentral scotoma. As with other psychophysical tests, the reliability of the Amsler grid test depends on patient comprehension and

cooperation. Other effective methods for assessing the central field are Goldmann perimetry (using the smallest visible stimulus), central automated fields like the Humphrey 20–10 or Octopus M2 and the tangent screen.

Diagnosis: Small homonymous scotoma due to occipital stroke

Tip: A small homonymous hemianopic scotoma can often be suspected from the history. The Amsler grid is a quick and effective method for assessing the central visual field in such cases.

Post-cardiac bypass visual loss

Case: A 63-year-old machinist experienced bilateral visual loss upon awakening after coronary artery bypass surgery. Visual acuity was 20/200 OU with markedly decreased color vision. By confrontation he appeared to have bilateral central scotomas, stating that he could see the examiner's hair, chin and ears but not eyes, nose and mouth. Ischemic optic neuropathy was suspected but the pupillary responses and optic disc appearance were normal.

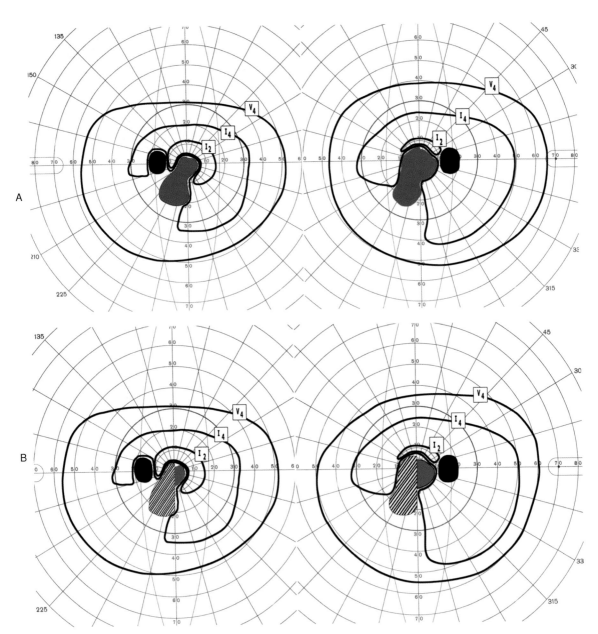

Figure 8.9 Goldmann perimetry in the above patient with bilateral visual loss following cardiac surgery. (A) His initial visual field was interpreted as showing bilateral central scotomas. (B) On closer inspection, these defects are actually bilateral homonymous hemianopic scotomas with a small mismatch along the vertical meridian.

Is there another possible explanation for this patient's visual loss, and how would you investigate this alternative mechanism?

Infarction of the retrobulbar segment of the optic nerves, called posterior ischemic optic neuropathy, would be consistent with a normal fundus appearance acutely. However, the presence of brisk pupil reflexes is not. The combination of marked bilateral central visual loss and normal pupillary responses suggests cortical visual loss, specifically due to a lesion involving the occipital tips. Initial examination of the field with Goldmann perimetry suggested bilateral central scotomas with an odd vertically ovoid shape (Figure 8.9A). Based on this appearance and the other clinical features, the central portion of the field was tested again, this time including careful exploration of the vertical meridian to either side of fixation. With this technique it was found that what appeared to be bilateral central scotomas were indeed matched, bilateral, homonymous hemianopic scotomas in the central field with a small vertical step between the two sides (Figure 8.9B). As expected based on the clinical findings, a CT scan revealed bilateral infarcts at the occipital tips (Figure 8.10). Based on the clinical context and radiographic appearance, the mechanism was presumed to be embolic.

Discussion: The topographic representation of information carried in the afferent visual pathways is displayed within the occipital cortex in a very precise arrangement. The central (macular) visual field is transmitted to the posterior aspect of the occipital lobes, also termed the "occipital tip". Information from the peripheral field is displayed more anteriorly, adjacent to the genu of the corpus callosum. The occipital lobes are separated by the interhemispheric fissure, and each receives its own blood supply. While damage to the occipital tips can produce bilateral homonymous defects, it is unlikely that the right and left defects would be perfectly symmetric. The resultant scotomas, therefore, show a mismatch along the vertical meridian, as in the above case. Because the posterior cerebral

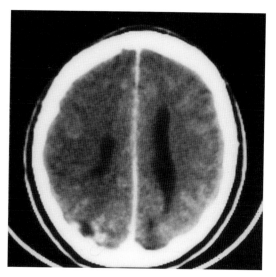

Figure 8.10 Axial post-contrast CT of the head shows areas of low density at the occipital tip bilaterally with adjacent gyriform enhancement on the right side.

arteries that supply the occipital lobes arise from a common trunk, the basilar artery, it is not uncommon for emboli traveling in this arterial system to arrive in both occipital lobes.

Although a *unilateral* post-geniculate lesion never affects visual acuity (still normal in the intact hemifield), a bilateral lesion involving macular fibers does produce loss of acuity of varying degree that is always symmetric in the two eyes. The resultant bilateral central visual loss often suggests bilateral optic neuropathy or maculopathy as the cause, and the finding of bilateral central scotomas furthers this impression. In such cases, careful inspection of the contours of the central scotomas, with particular attention to each side of the vertical meridian, should provide the correct localization. Goldmann perimetry is particularly well suited for such exploration but an automated field that concentrates on the central field, such as the Humphrey 10–2 program, should also provide comparable information.

Diagnosis: Bilateral homonymous hemianopic scotomas secondary to bilateral occipital tip strokes

Tip: Lesions at the occipital tips bilaterally can mimic bilateral optic neuropathy. Careful perimetry looking for a vertical mismatch should be diagnostic.

Pseudo-bitemporal defects

Optic nerve fibers originating in the nasal retina and serving the temporal visual field decussate at the optic chiasm. This anatomic fact explains the most common pattern of visual loss associated with a chiasmal lesion: a bitemporal hemianopia. There is no other place in the visual pathway where a single lesion can cause bilateral, non-homonymous visual field loss, and thus the presence of a bitemporal visual field defect that respects the vertical meridian is absolutely localizing to the optic chiasm (Figure 8.11). In principle, this concept is clear; in practice it is sometimes less straightforward.

Certain ocular conditions, when bilateral, can cause simultaneous temporal field losses. These include papilledema (bilaterally enlarged physiologic blindspots), disorders of the outer retina termed "big blindspot syndromes", retinal degenerations, macular disease, congenital disc anomalies and glaucoma. The bitemporal visual field defect found in these *ocular* disorders does not strictly respect the vertical meridian and is sometimes referred to as a *pseudo-bitemporal hemianopia*. Clinicians should be able to distinguish between a pseudo-bitemporal and a true bitemporal hemianopia in order to correctly localize the visual loss to the eye or to the chiasm. The following three cases highlight clues that are helpful in making this distinction.

Incidental field defect

Case: This 45-year-old librarian described a one-year history of difficulty reading, and gradual blurring of vision in both eyes. Her past medical history was significant only for pre-eclampsia during her

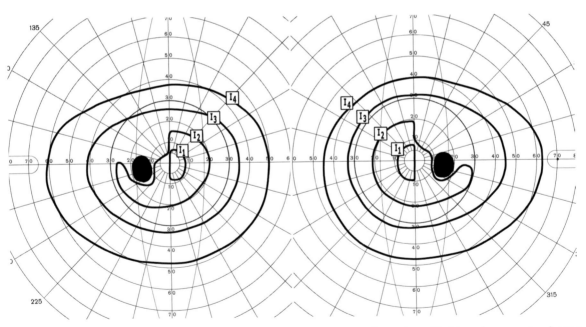

Figure 8.11 A bitemporal defect as demonstrated by Goldmann perimetry in a patient with chiasmal compression due to a pituitary tumor. Notice that the defect lines up along ("respects") the vertical meridian.

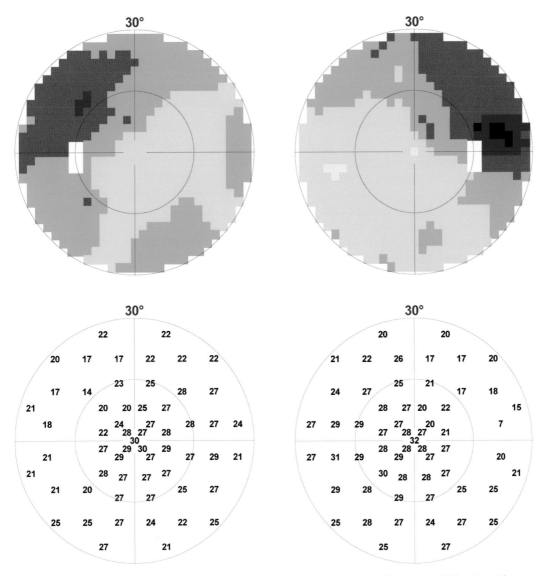

Figure 8.12 Central 26 degree automated threshold test (Octopus 101, G1 program) of a 45-year-old librarian with progressive difficulty reading due to presbyopia. The color scale and threshold values in decibel units are displayed. For interpretation, note that the higher the number, the dimmer the stimulus seen and the greater the visual sensitivity. There is focal visual loss (green-brown shading and lower threshold values) in the temporal hemifield of each eye, more marked superiorly.

last pregnancy five years ago. On examination, she was found to be presbyopic and her reading problems were alleviated with over-the-counter readers. A routine visual field test was also performed (Octopus 101, Interzeag AG, Bern, Switzerland), and rather unexpectedly the results were not normal (Figure 8.12). The remainder of her examination was unremarkable.

The visual field appeared to show a superior bitemporal hemianopia, suggesting the possibility of a chiasmal lesion. The patient underwent an MRI of brain and orbits which showed no abnormalities in the sellar region.

What is the next step in this patient's evaluation?

The issue at hand is whether or not this patient has chiasmal visual loss. Alignment of a temporal scotoma along the vertical meridian best distinguishes a chiasmal lesion from other conditions that produce similar field loss. In reviewing her automated test, we find that the individual threshold values show a clear temporal–nasal asymmetry across the vertical meridian superiorly, suggesting a true hemianopic defect; but there is also mildly decreased sensitivity that extends into the nasal field superiorly (green shading on the color scale representation). How accurately does the Octopus G1 program assess vertical alignment of a scotoma? The G1 measures the visual threshold at 59 loci within the central 26 degrees of visual field, and the loci are not evenly distributed throughout the field. At the foveal area, there are more test locations and the test points straddling the vertical meridian are very close to actual midline. With increasing eccentricity, the location of test points along the vertical meridian diverges, so that defining a true hemianopic border is less certain.

A more precise exploration of the vertical meridian is needed and there are several methods for accomplishing this. One is to select the automated program with a testing strategy specifically designed for this purpose, sometimes referred to as the "neuro program". Another option is testing with the Goldmann perimeter, paying particular attention to points on each side of the vertical meridian. A tangent screen is also effective for this purpose, with the patient seated one meter from the screen and tested with a small red target. In this case, the patient returned for Goldmann perimetry which demonstrated that the temporal scotomas actually extended into the adjacent nasal field, and thus represented a pseudo-bitemporal defect (Figure 8.13).

Based on the new interpretation of this patient's visual field defect, what feature of the examination should be reconsidered?

A more critical fundus examination revealed *tilted optic discs*, a congenital anomaly often associated with a pseudo-bitemporal hemianopic defect (Figure 8.14). The patient was reassured as to the benign nature of her visual field abnormality.

Discussion: The tilted disc is a congenital anomaly in which the superotemporal optic disc is elevated and the inferonasal disc is posteriorly displaced. The vertical axis of the disc is oriented obliquely, with angulation of the inferonasal aspect, which appears flattened and even hypoplastic. The tilted disc syndrome may include one or more associated findings: peri-papillary atrophy (scleral crescent), inferonasal chorioretinal hypoplasia and ectasia, and situs inversus of the retinal vessels. The degree of temporal field loss is variable and may appear as a scotoma or an area of depression. The field defect typically emerges from the physiologic blindspot, involves the superior temporal quadrant and, most importantly, crosses over into the superior nasal quadrant. The defect is at least in part refractive, due to ectasia of the inferonasal peri-papillary retina, which produces more myopia in this area compared to the surrounding retina. Consequently, the field defect can be reduced or even eliminated with the use of additional minus correction when testing that portion of the field. This disc anomaly often occurs in eyes with myopic astigmatism, is non-progressive and, unlike some other congenital ocular anomalies, is not associated with any abnormalities involving other organ systems.

Diagnosis: Tilted disc syndrome

Tip: Techniques that allow accurate assessment along the vertical meridian can distinguish chiasmal visual loss from other conditions that affect the temporal field.

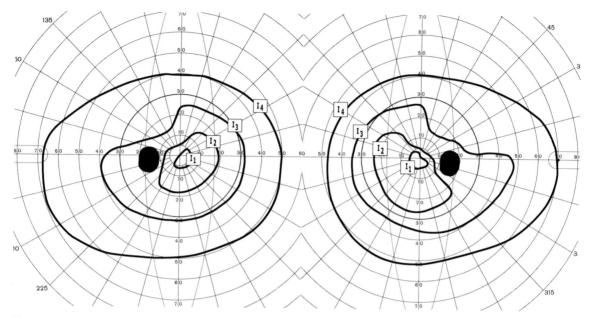

Figure 8.13 Goldmann perimetry in the above patient. This test confirms a defect in the superior temporal quadrant of each eye, but with this technique it is apparent that the defect slopes over the vertical meridian into the nasal hemifield.

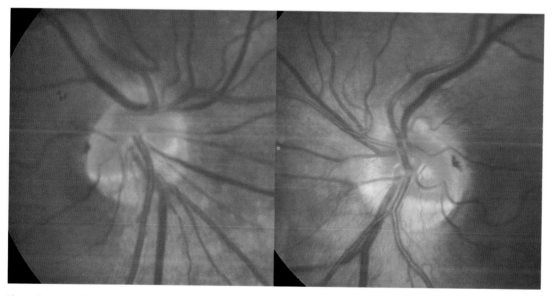

Figure 8.14 Fundus photographs of the above patient. The inferonasal aspect of each optic disc is truncated, producing a tilted disc configuration and adjacent peri-papillary pigment disturbance. In addition, the retinal vessels emerge nasally and then proceed temporally, termed "situs inversus."

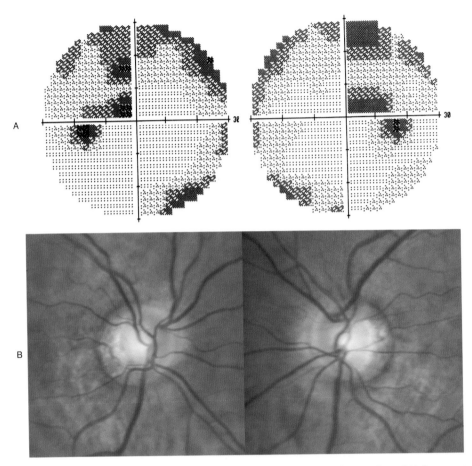

Figure 8.15 Visual testing in a visually asymptomatic 35-year-old homemaker. (A) Central 30 degree automated threshold perimetry (Humphrey Field Analyzer, 30–2, gray scale) shows a temporal scotoma in the superior field of each eye that appears to respect the vertical meridian. (B) Both optic discs are pale temporally.

Abnormal fields and temporal disc pallor

Case: A 35-year-old homemaker was referred for neuro-ophthalmic consultation because of abnormal visual fields found during a routine screening test. She had no visual symptoms, though she did recall having had some difficulty reading the eye chart at her last driver's examination but had passed nevertheless. She was generally healthy and took no medications. She was a non-smoker, consumed occasional alcohol and had a normal diet. Her family history included long-standing visual loss in a sister and in her father. Visual acuity was correctable to 20/25 in each eye, pupillary responses were normal and she identified 13 of 15 pseudoisochromatic plates OU. The optic discs were pale temporally and fundus examination was otherwise normal (Figure 8.15B). Humphrey perimetry (Zeiss-Humphrey, San Leandro, CA, USA) showed a superior temporal defect in each eye that appeared to respect the vertical meridian (Figure 8.15A). This visual field pattern suggested a lesion involving the optic chiasm, however a high quality MRI of this area was completely normal.

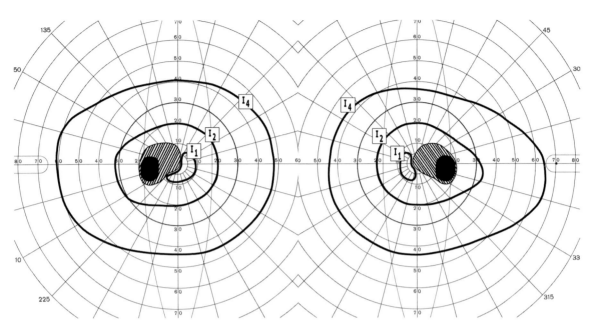

Figure 8.16 Goldmann perimetry in the same patient demonstrates a defect emerging from the physiologic blindspot and extending toward fixation in each eye (bilateral ceco-central scotomas).

The visual fields were re-assessed using Goldmann perimetry (Figure 8.16). Note that the parafoveal scotomas are fairly dense but the mid-peripheral and peripheral isopters are intact and do not demonstrate a superotemporal vertical step. The scotomas encroach on the smallest isopter in each eye but do not align along the vertical meridian. With this testing technique it is apparent that the defects are actually ceco-central scotomas that just happen to abut close to the vertical meridian. In light of this new interpretation of the visual field pattern, and in conjunction with the other clinical features, a diagnosis of dominant (Kjer's) optic atrophy was considered. Records regarding other family members were obtained and were found to be consistent with this diagnosis.

Discussion: *Dominant optic atrophy* is a form of progressive optic neuropathy inherited in an autosomal dominant fashion but with variable penetrance. The responsible mutation has been localized to the OP1 A gene, but the nature of the mutation varies among affected families. Onset of symptoms typically begins by age 10 and progresses very slowly over a lifetime. Central vision is predominantly affected, including loss of color vision with a characteristic tritanopic (blue-yellow) axis pattern. The optic discs show temporal pallor, which is sometimes accompanied by focal excavation. The degree of visual loss exhibits marked inter-individual variability, even among members of the same family. At the mild end of the spectrum some affected individuals retain 20/20 visual acuity and may therefore be unaware of their diagnosis. In suspected cases it may be helpful to actually examine relatives rather than relying on the patient's report of a negative family history.

Diagnosis: Dominant optic atrophy

Tip: Bilateral ceco-central scotomas that abut the vertical meridian may mimic a chiasmal pattern of field loss, particularly on automated perimetry.

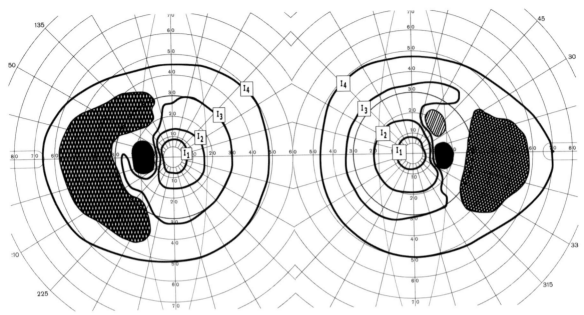

Figure 8.17 Goldmann perimetry in a 64-year-old homemaker with photopsias and nyctalopia. There is a large, dense scotoma in the peripheral and mid-peripheral temporal field of each eye, largely sparing central isopters.

Abnormal field and photopsias

Case: A 64-year-old homemaker was referred because of a five-year history of persistent photopsias. She had also noted some difficulty seeing in dim illumination, such as finding her way in a darkened movie theater. She was generally healthy and family history was negative for similar visual loss. Examination showed normal visual acuity, color vision and pupillary responses. Goldmann perimetry demonstrated a dense scotoma in the temporal field of each eye (Figure 8.17). An MR scan was obtained, specifically looking for chiasmal compression, but was completely normal.

What aspect of this patient's visual field defect is atypical for chiasmal compression and suggests instead an ocular disorder?

Her bitemporal defect involves the periphery and mid-periphery of the visual field, sparing the centralmost area. This pattern of field loss suggests a disorder of photoreceptors rather than an

optic nerve or chiasmal lesion. In addition, while the defects are indeed confined to the temporal hemifield of each eye, they do not respect the vertical meridian. This patient had a full-field ERG that demonstrated marked loss of scotopic waveforms with mild reduction of photopic responses, consistent with a rod-cone dystrophy (Figure 8.18).

Discussion: About 90% of axons in the optic nerves and chiasm subserve the central 10 degrees of the visual field. Therefore, the earliest visual field change in chiasmal compression involves macular vision, usually appearing as a small, shallow defect just temporal (often superotemporal) to fixation in each eye. With continued compression, the central hemianopic defect grows in size and density, eventually breaking out to the periphery. This predilection for central field loss in chiasmal compression is in marked contrast to the pattern of loss seen in the above patient whose bitemporal defect was most marked in the mid-periphery. This pattern should suggest, instead, a retinal disorder, specifically one involving photoreceptors. The diagnosis of retinal

A

B

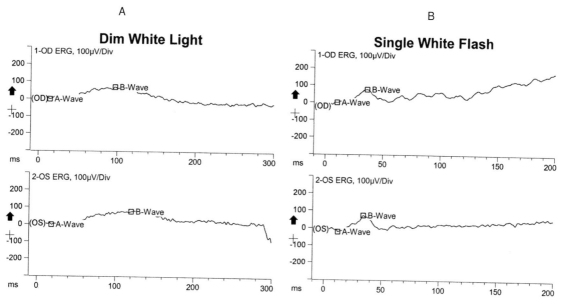

Figure 8.18 Full-field ERG of both eyes in the above patient. (A) Under scotopic conditions there is moderate loss of b-wave amplitude in each eye. (B) Under photopic conditions, the b-wave amplitude in each eye is only mildly diminished.

dystrophy was confirmed by the results of her ERG. This patient's history of nyctalopia and photopsias was also consistent with the diagnosis of photoreceptor disease.

Diagnosis: Rod-cone dystrophy

Tip: Bitemporal defects due to chiasmal compression preferentially involve the central field because macular fibers are affected early and most prominently. Defects demonstrating the opposite pattern, i.e. central sparing, should suggest a retinal disorder.

FURTHER READING

Visual field testing

D. R. Anderson, *Perimetry, With and Without Automation*, 2nd edn. St. Louis: Mosby, 1987.

D. R. Anderson, *Automated Static Perimetry*. St. Louis: Mosby, 1992.

D. O. Harrington, *The Visual Fields. A Textbook and Atlas of Clinical Perimetry*, 5th edn. St. Louis: Mosby, 1981.

Tilted disc syndrome

P. D. Brazitikos, A. B. Safran, F. Simona, M. Zulauf, Threshold perimetry in tilted disc syndrome. *Arch Ophthalmol*, **108** (1990), 1698–1700.

M. C. Brodsky, Congenital optic disk anomalies. *Surv Ophthalmol*, **39** (1994), 89–112.

L. Manfré, S. Vero, C. Focarelli-Baronne, R. Lagaua, Bitemporal pseudohemianopia related to the "tilted disk" syndrome: CT, MR, and funduscopic findings. *AJNR Am J Neuroradiol*, **20** (1999), 1750–1.

Dominant optic atrophy

D. Eliott, E. I. Traboulsi, I. H. Maumenee, Visual prognosis in autosomal dominant optic atrophy (Kjer type). *Am J Ophthalmol*, **115** (1993), 360–7.

C. S. Hoyt, Autosomal dominant optic atrophy. A spectrum of disability. *Ophthalmology*, **87** (1980), 245–51.

R. L. Johnston, M. J. Seller, J. T. Benham, M. A. Burdon, D. J. Spalton, Dominant optic atrophy: Refining the clinical diagnostic criteria in light of genetic linkage studies. *Ophthalmology*, **106** (1999), 123–8.

9

Neuro-ophthalmic look-alikes

In every-day clinical practice, there are usually a number of disorders that could account for a particular presentation, and our job is to distinguish among them. In this chapter, however, we will focus on cases in which there are just two main diagnostic possibilities, and look at how these two conditions are distinguished. For teaching purposes, we will highlight the *one* best feature that differentiates the two disorders in question. The main point of this chapter is to provide the clinician with specific tips on how to distinguish between two common "look-alike" diagnoses.

Idiopathic optic neuritis vs. Leber's hereditary optic neuropathy

Case: A 35-year-old accountant noted rapidly progressive visual loss in his left eye, described as a "bright fog", which developed over a 10-day period. Examination revealed visual acuity of 20/400 OS, a moderate (2+) left RAPD and dense central scotoma (Figure 9.1A). The right optic disc had a normal appearance, the left optic disc was slightly swollen and just a bit hyperemic. The remainder of the fundus examination was unremarkable (Figure 9.1B). The patient was in good general health and taking no medications. He had no history of prior neurologic deficits and his family history was negative for neurologic or eye disease.

Based on this patient's clinical presentation, what is your first diagnostic consideration?

Acute onset of unilateral optic neuropathy in a young adult is most often due to idiopathic

(demyelinating) optic neuritis. A predilection for central visual loss is typical, as in the above case. In the acute stage, the optic disc is either swollen (in one-third of patients) or normal. This patient had an MRI of brain and orbits including contrast administration, which was completely normal, and then received a course of IV methylprednisolone for a presumptive diagnosis of isolated idiopathic optic neuritis. He was assured that most patients with this diagnosis experience recovery of vision to 20/40 or better. His vision, however, did not show the expected improvement and eight weeks later he noticed onset of similar visual loss in the fellow eye.

Does his clinical course change your mind about the diagnosis?

Lack of visual improvement by four to six weeks after onset is so atypical for idiopathic optic neuritis that other causes of optic neuropathy must be investigated. In this case, failure to recover vision in the affected eye, plus the early development of similar visual loss in the second eye, pointed to the alternative diagnosis of Leber's hereditary optic neuropathy (LHON). Molecular genetic testing of this patient's mitochondrial DNA revealed a point mutation at 11778, termed the Wallace mutation, confirming a diagnosis of LHON.

Was there a "red flag" at the time of his *initial* presentation?

Absence of pain at the onset of this patient's visual loss would be highly atypical for idiopathic optic

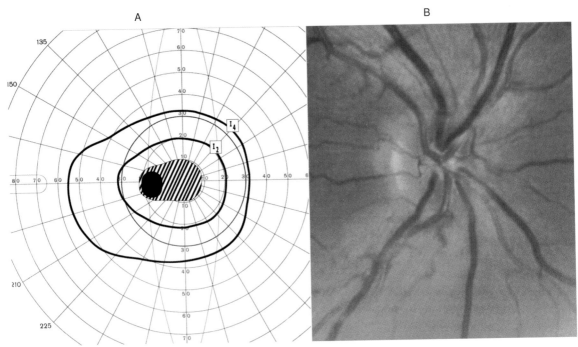

Figure 9.1 Examination findings in a 35-year-old accountant with recent painless visual loss in the left eye. (A) Goldmann perimetry in the left eye shows a dense ceco-central scotoma. (B) There is mild fullness and hyperemia of the left disc.

neuritis. More than 90% of patients with idiopathic optic neuritis experience ipsilateral eye pain, usually exacerbated by eye movement and accompanied by globe tenderness. In a patient who seems to have optic neuritis but without pain, it is important to consider alternative possibilities, including ischemic optic neuropathy, neuroretinitis, compressive optic neuropathy, a variety of maculopathies and LHON. In retrospect, the normal orbital MRI should also have cast some doubt on the diagnosis of optic neuritis; abnormal optic nerve enhancement is present in approximately 90% of cases.

Discussion: *Leber's hereditary optic neuropathy* (LHON) is characterized by acute to subacute onset of painless central visual loss. The usual age at onset is between 15 and 35 years, hence the overlapping profile with idiopathic optic neuritis. LHON has a strong male preponderance (80–90%) in contrast to the female predilection in optic neu-

ritis (approximately 75%), so this patient's gender alone is grounds for considering an alternative diagnosis, particularly LHON. Visual loss usually occurs sequentially and deteriorates over several months before stabilization. Second eye involvement occurs in most cases within weeks to months after the first eye. As in the above case, visual loss is often attributed to optic neuritis initially but when the second eye is affected the diagnosis of LHON becomes apparent.

Optic disc appearance in LHON is variable. Some patients exhibit apparent hyperemic swelling of the disc. What appear to be dilated capillaries on the disc surface actually represent a fine network of vessels referred to as *circumpapillary telangiectatic microangiopathy*, or, alternatively, *peri-papillary microvascular angiopathy*. These vessels can be distinguished from other forms of disc hyperemia by their failure to show leakage on fluorescein angiography. Accompanying the microangiopathy is a thickened appearance of the nerve fiber layer, termed "*pseudo-edema*". This characteristic fundus appearance may be present prior to the onset of visual loss and can also be seen in about half of unaffected family members, many of whom never progress to visual loss. In about one-third of patients with symptomatic LHON, the disc has a completely normal appearance at the time of initial visual loss. Hence, a normal fundus appearance in no way rules out a diagnosis of LHON. In some cases, optic atrophy has already developed by the time the patient is evaluated.

LHON is a maternally inherited disorder due to a point mutation in the mitochondrial DNA complex I genes. Four mutations (11778, 3460, 14484 and 14459) are considered "primary" and account for approximately 95% of cases, with the 11778 mutation alone accounting for about 50%. A fifth, 15257, may be another primary LHON mutation but is also found in low frequency in control groups. Genetic testing is strongly recommended, not only for diagnostic confirmation, but also for prognostic value. In most patients with symptomatic LHON, visual loss is usually profound and permanent. Yet an occasional patient experiences some degree of spontaneous improvement and the likelihood of such recovery is related to the specific mutation. Only 4% of patients with the common 11778 mutation experience visual improvement, whereas the other mutations are associated with a higher percentage of spontaneous visual recovery. The onset of visual recovery, when it does occur, can be surprisingly delayed, occurring from three months to several years after initial visual loss.

There is currently no effective treatment for visual loss due to LHON. Exogenous factors such as systemic infection, nutritional deficiency, medications and exposure to toxins have been explored as possible triggers that may provoke the onset or increase the risk of phenotypic expression, but no definite causal relationship has been confirmed for any of these. Nonetheless, patients who harbor a LHON mutation are strongly advised to discontinue smoking, avoid exposure to solvents and other fumes and take daily vitamin supplements.

Genetic counselling is an important aspect of management in patients with LHON. Phenotypic penetrance of the LHON mutation is notably incomplete; many individuals carry the mutation but never suffer visual loss. Because all mitochondria are maternally inherited, men with the LHON mutation never pass on the disorder and male patients should be assured of this fact. However, all female relatives of a male proband are obligatory carriers, and will necessarily transmit the mutation to all their children. In addition to being carriers, 5 to 20% of females with a primary LHON mutation will eventually experience visual loss. In contrast, male carriers have a much greater lifetime risk of visual loss, ranging from 25 to 60%. The basis for this gender-specific susceptibility is unknown.

Since the availability of genetic testing for this disorder, our understanding of the clinical features has greatly expanded, including confirmed cases of LHON occurring in young children and in individuals over age 65 years. Atypical temporal patterns have also been described, including sudden bilateral blindness and protracted visual deterioration over years. These variations in the phenotype serve as reminders that LHON should be included in the differential diagnosis of any patient with an acute painless optic neuropathy, regardless of age and gender.

The clinical scenario: Acute monocular optic neuropathy with central visual loss in a young adult

The look-alikes: Idiopathic optic neuritis vs. Leber's hereditary optic neuropathy

Tip: Absence of pain, male gender and normal MRI strongly suggest the possibility of Leber's hereditary optic neuropathy.

Acute tonic pupil vs. pharmacologic mydriasis

Case: A 40-year-old oncology nurse accidently splashed disinfecting solution in his right eye while cleaning a countertop. He immediately experienced a burning sensation and copiously lavaged his eye.

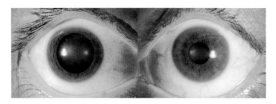

Figure 9.2 Pupils of the above nurse with accidental chemical exposure to the right eye three days earlier. The right pupil is markedly dilated and unresponsive to light stimulation and near effort; the left pupil is normal in shape, size and reactivity.

Several days later, he noted photophobia, blurred vision and a dilated pupil on that side (Figure 9.2).

Examination three days later revealed normal visual acuities at distance, but near vision in his right eye was poor (about 20/200) and required a +3.00 lens to achieve 20/20. In room light, his right pupil measured 8 mm and appeared to be completely unreactive to direct and consensual light stimulation. The left pupil measured 4 mm and had a normal light reflex. When the patient was asked to focus on a near object, there was normal convergence and pupillary constriction on the left side but there was no change in the right pupil. Ocular motility and fundus appearance were normal bilaterally. The anterior chamber was quiet and intraocular pressures were normal.

What common mechanisms of injury could explain this patient's pupillary dysfunction?

A dilated pupil that does not constrict to light stimulation or to near effort indicates impairment of the iris sphincter. Possible mechanisms include direct damage to the sphincter muscle, pharmacologic paralysis of sphincter activity or denervation. In this case, there was no history of ocular trauma or prior surgery and the iris appeared structurally intact. The accidental chemical exposure to the eye in question raised the possibility of pharmacologic pupillary dilation. It was assumed that the disinfecting solution must have contained a parasympatholytic (atropine-like) agent that blocked the postsynaptic

receptors on the sphincter muscle. Thus, a diagnosis of pharmacologic mydriasis was made. The patient was told that his pupil should soon return to normal. Three weeks later, however, his examination was unchanged and therefore the possibility of postganglionic parasympathetic denervation of the sphincter was entertained.

What examination finding can distinguish pharmacologic blockade from postganglionic denervation of the iris sphincter?

Sectoral palsy, visible as a demarcation between areas of functioning and non-functioning iris sphincter, rules out pharmacologic blockade and localizes the site of damage instead to the peripheral short ciliary nerves. This is because pharmacologic agents, e.g. atropine-like substances, act diffusely on the iris sphincter and cannot produce sectoral paralysis. Slit-lamp examination with high magnification showed that this patient's right iris sphincter was not completely paralyzed. There was a small nasal segment (between the two and four o'clock segments) that demonstrated normal contractility (Figure 9.3). General medical and neurologic examinations were otherwise normal as were blood glucose, general chemistries, syphilis serology and an erythrocyte sedimentation rate. A diagnosis of acute, idiopathic tonic (Adie's) pupil was made. The close temporal relationship between the onset of his tonic pupil and the chemical exposure turned out to be purely coincidental. At two-month follow-up, his right pupil was still dilated and poorly reactive to light but now demonstrated cholinergic supersensitivity and light-near dissociation.

Discussion: Acute postganglionic denervation of the iris sphincter (Adie's tonic pupil) and ocular exposure to an atropine-like agent can both lead to a large pupil, on the order of 7–9 mm in room light, that is unresponsive to light and near stimulation. Over time, a denervated pupil often develops cholinergic supersensitivity, light-near dissociation, and tonicity, but these characteristic features of an Adie's pupil are not present in the first week (see also

A   B

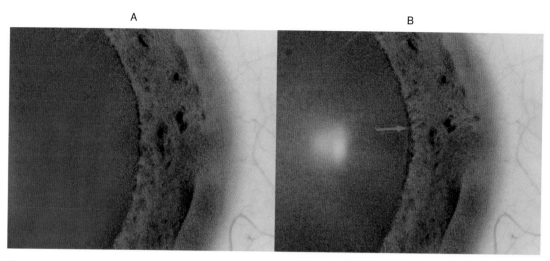

Figure 9.3 Right pupillary sphincter (nasal margin) of the above patient viewed at high magnification with the slit-lamp. (A) The iris stroma appears flat and the pupillary ruff is thin. (B) With bright light stimulation, the entire sphincter remains immobile except for a small area nasally. This contractile segment produces a few folds of iris and the adjacent pupillary ruff becomes denser and thicker (arrow).

Chapter 11, Isolated unilateral mydriasis). Thus, in the acute state, the only examination feature that effectively distinguishes denervation injury and pharmacologic mydriasis is the presence of *sectoral palsy of the iris sphincter*. An acutely denervated pupil may appear to have no light reflex when observed with the unaided eye. However, under high magnification at the slit-lamp or by using a magnifying glass and a bright hand-held light source, sectoral sphincter palsy is almost always visible. Sectoral palsy is detected by carefully watching each clock-hour segment of the sphincter as the illuminator light is rapidly turned on and off. Paralyzed sectors of the sphincter have an absent or thinned pupillary ruff, and the contour of the pupillary margin appears flattened (Figure 9.4). In addition, the iris segment adjacent to the palsied sector makes a characteristic undulating movement when the light is turned on, termed stromal streaming, due to passive pulling of the stroma toward normally contracting segments of iris.

Sectoral sphincter palsy is highly suggestive of, but not limited to, peripheral nerve injury. Direct injury to the iris can result in similar focal paralysis of the sphincter muscle. In such cases, however, there is usually a history of trauma, intraocular inflammation or ocular surgery, as well as visible evidence of damage to other anterior segment structures. When it is unclear if the site of injury is the muscle or the nerve, look for other signs of postganglionic nerve injury such as cholinergic supersensitivity, light-near dissociation and tonicity, which favor a diagnosis of tonic pupil.

Sectoral sphincter palsy persists in the chronic phase of an Adie's pupil and remains an extremely valuable clinical feature. While clinicians often depend on the dilute pilocarpine test to confirm a diagnosis of Adie's pupil, it is important to remember that the demonstration of cholinergic supersensitivity using dilute pilocarpine is neither completely sensitive nor specific. About 20% of patients with tonic pupils fail to demonstrate such enhanced sensitivity. More importantly, cholinergic supersensitivity is also present in some patients with disruption of the preganglionic parasympathetic impulses to the iris, i.e. a third nerve palsy. The diagnosis of an Adie's pupil is most confidently based on a constellation of clinical findings, the

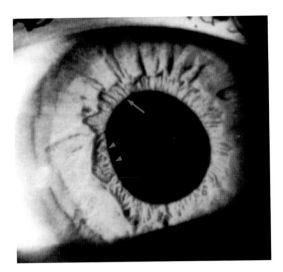

Figure 9.4 Close-up view of a right Adie's pupil in a different patient. There is sectoral palsy involving the inferotemporal aspect of the sphincter, which produces thinning of the iris stroma and flattening of the pupillary margin between 7:00 and 10:00 (arrowheads). Adjacent to this paralyzed sector is a normally innervated segment of sphincter (11:00 to 12:00) where the iris stroma "bunches up" like a pulled purse string and the pupillary margin rounds out (arrow). (From H. S. Thompson, Segmental palsy of the iris sphincter in Adie's syndrome. *Arch Ophthalmol*, **96** (1978), 1615–20, with permission.)

most reassuring of which is the presence of sectoral palsy.

The clinical scenario: Acute, isolated unilateral mydriasis

The look-alikes: Pharmacologic mydriasis vs. acute Adie's tonic pupil

Tip: Sectoral sphincter palsy is found in tonic pupils but not in pharmacologic pupillary dilation.

Chronic tonic pupils vs. Argyll Robertson pupils

Case: A 75-year-old woman was referred by her internist for evaluation of small pupils that did not react to light. She was not using any systemic or top-

ical medications known to constrict pupils. Visual acuity was 20/20 in each eye and confrontation fields were normal. In room light, her pupils measured 2.5 mm and were not appreciably larger in dim lighting. There was no response of either pupil to a bright light. When the patient was asked to focus on a near target, however, both pupils constricted (Figure 9.5). The remainder of her neurologic examination was normal and a VDRL (Venereal Disease Research Laboratory) test was negative.

This patient's internist was concerned that her small, poorly reactive pupils with light-near dissociation (LND) might indicate late neurosyphilis. The alternative diagnosis of chronic bilateral Adie's pupils should also be considered, however. While

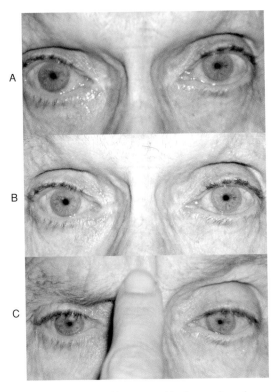

Figure 9.5 A 75-year-old woman with abnormal pupils. (A) In dim illumination the pupils are small and equal in size. With bright light stimulation (B) there is no noticeable change in pupillary size, but with near effort (C) both pupils constrict.

an acute Adie's tonic pupil is large, over time its size tends to diminish. The mechanism for this change is related to the amount of aberrant re-innervation of the iris sphincter that is characteristic of this syndrome. Accommodative fibers, unlike pupillary fibers, normally release a constant volley of discharges, which leads to a state of tonic sphincter contraction. As progressively more accommodative fibers regenerate, they innervate more segments of the iris sphincter, causing these segments to become chronically contracted. This leads to a progressively smaller baseline pupil size, sometimes referred to as a "little old Adie's". In contrast, the relative paucity of regenerating pupillomotor fibers means that the light reflex remains poor, regardless of pupillary size. In addition, there is a tendency for the fellow pupil to become similarly involved so that about half of patients with an Adie's pupil develop bilateral involvement by 10 years. As a result of these two features, long-standing Adie's pupils may easily be mistaken for syphilitic pupils, as in the above case.

Is there a physical finding that can differentiate chronic Adie's pupils from Argyll Robertson pupils?

The *speed* of the pupillary movement is an important differential feature in eyes with LND. Tonic pupils have a delayed, slow constriction to near effort and, more importantly, also demonstrate sustained constriction and a similarly slow re-dilation upon distance refixation. In contrast, Argyll Robertson pupils constrict to near effort with the briskness of normally innervated pupils and promptly re-dilate after release of near effort. In this patient, pupillary constriction during near effort was extremely slow, as was pupillary dilation upon refixation to a distant target. This finding of delayed, slow and sustained pupillary movement points to a diagnosis of tonic pupils.

Discussion: The chief abnormality in this patient is pupillary light-near dissociation (LND). Individuals who are blind due to disease of the anterior

visual pathways have little or no pupil light reflex, but their pupil near reflex, stimulated by the intention to fixate a near target, is intact. Blindness is actually the most common cause of LND, but it rarely poses any diagnostic confusion. In patients with normal vision, LND is often due to dorsal midbrain damage, sometimes considered a "central" mechanism of LND. The Edinger–Westphal nucleus is the main pupillomotor center and receives afferent input from a variety of sources. Afferent signals arising from the dorsal midbrain and the periaqueductal region mediate the *pupil light reflex*. In contrast, afferent signals mediating the *pupillary near response* approach the Edinger–Westphal nucleus ventrally (Figure 9.6). Central LND results from an injury to the midbrain that selectively interrupts the more dorsally situated fibers mediating the pupil light reflex pathway but spares the ventrally located fibers that mediate the near reflex. The most common causes of central LND are stroke, pineal tumors and hydrocephalus (see Chapter 10, Upgaze palsy). In most of these cases, the pupillary abnormality is accompanied by other deficits related to dorsal midbrain dysfunction, including upgaze palsy, lid retraction, skew deviation and convergence-retraction nystagmus (Parinaud's syndrome). The exact mechanism of the LND in tertiary syphilis (Argyll Robertson pupils) is not fully understood, but likely shares a similar mechanism involving selective de-afferentation of the pupillomotor center due to periaqueductal inflammation and gliosis.

A completely different mechanism underlies the light-near dissociation seen with tonic pupils (see above, Acute tonic pupil vs. pharmacologic mydriasis). The initial event is acute injury to the short ciliary nerves, the fibers that carry postganglionic parasympathetic impulses to the iris sphincter and ciliary body. Thereafter, typical of peripheral nerve injury, the short ciliary nerves begin to resprout. However, the short ciliary nerves contain a far greater number of accommodative fibers compared to pupil fibers so in the process of regeneration and reinnervation, the iris sphincter becomes increasingly innervated with accommodative fibers. In this

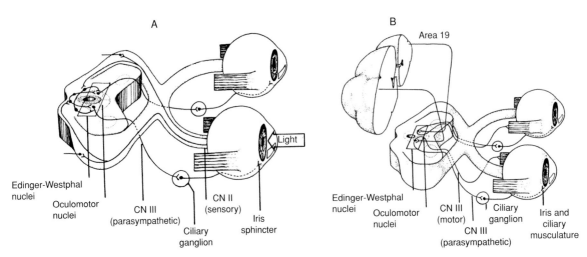

Figure 9.6 Pathways for the pupillary light reflex (A) and near reflex (B). Note that input to the Edinger–Westphal nuclei for the light reflex passes through the dorsal midbrain, whereas for the near response the approach is ventral to the aqueduct.

fashion, the pupil near response is restored, but the pupil light reflex remains absent or dysfunctional. Thus, the peripheral form of LND is due to aberrant regeneration bringing restoration of the near reflex whereas central LND is due dorsal midbrain injury impairing the light reflex while sparing the near reflex.

The clinical scenario: Bilaterally small pupils with light-near dissociation

The look-alikes: Chronic Adie's pupils vs. Argyll Robertson pupils

Tip: In a patient with pupillary light-near dissociation, slow and sustained contraction of the sphincter during and after near effort is characteristic of an Adie's pupil.

Convergence spasm vs. bilateral sixth nerve palsies

Case: A 23-year-old girl was referred because of a two-week history of diplopia, frontal headaches and blurred vision. Her diplopia was horizontal and intermittent, worse at distance than at near, and

present in all fields of gaze. She was taking no medications and there was no history of trauma. Visual acuity was 20/100 at distance in each eye. Confrontation visual fields and fundus appearance were normal and there was no ptosis or proptosis. She was esotropic in primary position but the angle of esodeviation varied during cross-cover testing. There was moderate limitation of abduction in both eyes that was also variable (Figure 9.7). The remainder of her neurologic examination was normal. Bilateral sixth nerve palsy was diagnosed and the patient was referred for immediate neuro-imaging.

While the presence of esotropia and abduction deficits suggests a diagnosis of bilateral sixth nerve palsy, the marked variability of her abduction deficit raised the possibility of myasthenia or convergence spasm.

What clinical findings would support a diagnosis of convergence spasm?

The key to making this diagnosis, also termed *spasm of the near reflex,* is the presence of other components of the near triad during periods of ocular misalignment. This is usually demonstrated by

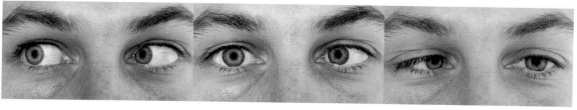

Figure 9.7 Motility examination in a 23-year-old girl with intermittent diplopia and headaches. In primary position there is moderate esotropia. On lateral gaze to each side there is limitation of abduction, mild in the right eye and more marked in the left.

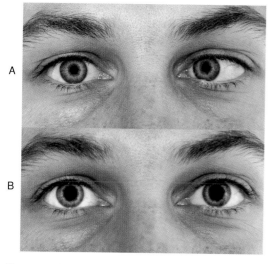

Figure 9.8 The same patient seen during an episode of esotropia (A) and between episodes when the eyes were aligned (B). Note that pupillary constriction accompanies the esotropia.

observing constriction of the pupils during episodes of esotropia. Closer examination in this patient did reveal marked miosis during periods of esotropia (Figure 9.8). Further history disclosed that her symptoms began shortly after the unexpected death of a family member. She was reassured as to the benign nature of this condition and six months later her examination was completely normal.

In addition to pupillary constriction during episodes of esotropia, excessive contraction of the ciliary body is also present, accounting for blurred vision at distance in this syndrome. The degree of

such accommodative spasm depends in large part on the age of the patient. In children and young adults, the resultant *pseudomyopia*, demonstrated by a disparity between the manifest and cycloplegic refractions, can be quite large.

Another helpful examination technique for identifying convergence spasm is comparison of ocular motility with binocular vs. monocular viewing. Tested with both eyes open, the patient with convergence spasm demonstrates variable esotropia and an apparent (usually bilateral) abduction deficit. When one eye is patched, the same patient will often demonstrate a strikingly normal range of abduction (Figure 9.9). In addition, there is often a disparity between eye movements when tested formally (refixation saccades and pursuit movements) versus performed during random eye movements. When convergence spasm is suspected, one should observe the patient's ocular motility while conversing or while performing other tasks.

Discussion: The near reflex is a normal synkinesis of convergence, accommodation and pupillary constriction that serves to keep a near target in focus on the fovea. Spasm of the near reflex occurs when this reflex is inappropriate for the visual task, i.e. invoked during distance fixation or excessively strong for a near target. Such spasm of the near reflex may occur as discrete episodes or, less commonly, as sustained activation of these three components. Symptoms include blurred vision, diplopia and brow ache. When convergence spasm is the prominent feature, episodic and variable esotropia may be mistaken for ocular myasthenia, but the

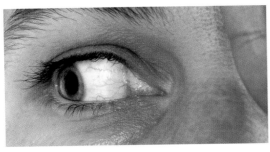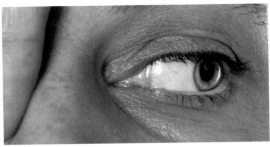

Figure 9.9 The same patient on right and then left gaze with the adducting eye patched. There is now full abduction in each eye with monocular viewing. Note also that the pupils are larger compared to Figure 9.8 when abduction was limited.

observation of miosis and/or pseudomyopia should distinguish spasm of the near reflex. Some patients also exhibit other excessive facial movements such as squinting, blinking or grimacing during episodes of esotropia. When convergence spasm is more sustained, persistent esotropia may be attributed to unilateral or bilateral sixth nerve palsy. Sixth nerve palsy is characterized by esotropia that worsens in lateral gaze and is greater at distance than near and, importantly, slowing of abduction saccades.

Unlike many brainstem reflexes which are unconscious and involuntary, the near reflex can be activated voluntarily. The large majority of cases of convergence spasm are functional in nature, i.e. non-organic. Rarely, spasm of the near reflex is due to organic disease and in such cases other neurologic abnormalities are typically present. These organic causes of convergence spasm include midbrain disorders (stroke, encephalitis and tumors), metabolic derangements (Wernicke's encephalopathy, phenytoin toxicity) and Chiari I malformation. Head trauma occasionally produces sustained accommodative spasm. In a neurologically intact patient with isolated, episodic convergence spasm, neuro-imaging is unnecessary. In patients with a history of head trauma, persistent spasm or other neurologic deficits, neuro-imaging and metabolic evaluation is recommended.

In the absence of an organic cause, management of patients with spasm of the near reflex is generally symptomatic. Diverse strategies are used but none with great success. Sources of stress and anxiety can often be identified and, ideally, corrected. Relax-

ation exercises such as meditation and yoga may be of some benefit. A variety of anxiolytic agents and muscle relaxants have been employed with varying results. It is sometimes tempting to prescribe refractive correction for the induced myopia, but this can be problematic because the patient is then required to maintain vigorous accommodation in order to see clearly. Alternatively, accommodative spasm can be blocked with a trial of topical cycloplegics, but the patient will then need reading glasses for near tasks. Furnishing base-out prism for convergence spasm is rarely helpful since the degree of esotropia is so variable.

The clinical scenario: Acute esotropia with bilateral abduction deficits

The look-alikes: Bilateral sixth nerve palsies vs. convergence spasm

Tip: Esotropia due to convergence spasm is accompanied by miosis.

Wernicke's encephalopathy vs. brainstem stroke

Case: A 39-year-old real estate agent was in the first trimester of her first pregnancy when she awoke with diplopia. She had not been well for several days, feeling lethargic, off-balance and slightly disoriented; symptoms that she attributed to severe morning sickness during the previous eight weeks. She was not taking any medications and had been

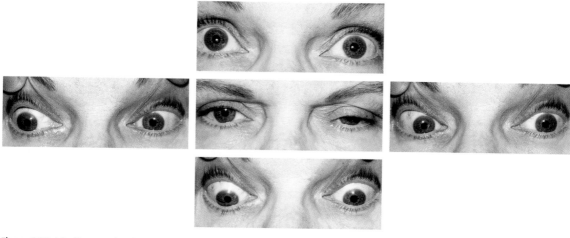

Figure 9.10 Motility examination in a 39-year-old pregnant woman with acute diplopia. There is bilateral ptosis, left greater than right, and moderate limitation of eye movements in all directions.

previously healthy. Examination revealed bilateral ptosis, limitation of gaze in all directions, slow upward saccades, upbeat nystagmus and mild ataxia (Figure 9.10). On cross-cover testing there was a small right hyperphoria. She was suspected of having suffered a brainstem stroke due to a pregnancy-related hypercoagulable state.

What aspect of this case makes an acute brainstem stroke unlikely?

This patient exhibits both horizontal *and* vertical gaze deficits. The center for horizontal conjugate gaze is the paramedian pontine reticular formation (PPRF) in the pons, whereas the structure that generates vertical saccades is the rostral interstitial nucleus of the medial longitudinal fasciculus (riMLF) in the midbrain. Therefore, this combination of ocular motor deficits cannot be explained by a single anatomic lesion. This patient must have either multiple brainstem lesions or a non-structural disease process.

What metabolic abnormality can produce this clinical picture?

Wernicke's encephalopathy is a neurologic syndrome caused by *thiamine (B1) deficiency* and characterized clinically by ophthalmoplegia, ataxia and confusion. The full triad, however, is present in only a minority of cases. It is therefore important to be able to recognize this condition based on parts of the complete syndrome. Ocular motility disturbance is the earliest and most constant finding in this disorder. Based on the patient's history of persistent vomiting, a presumptive diagnosis of Wernicke's encephalopathy was made. A brain MRI was normal. The patient was treated with 100 mg of thiamine intravenously and showed marked improvement of signs and symptoms within two to three days. She was discharged on anti-emetics and oral thiamine supplementation, and the remainder of her pregnancy was uneventful.

Discussion: *Wernicke's encephalopathy* is a preventable cause of neurologic morbidity in which prompt recognition and treatment directly influence the clinical outcome. The key to making this diagnosis is a high index of suspicion based on an awareness of the risk factors for thiamine depletion. These include persistent vomiting of any cause (e.g. hyperemesis gravidarum, gastrointestinal disorders or chemotherapy) and nutritional deficiency states such as chronic alcoholism, prolonged intravenous alimentation and malignancy (see Table 9.1). A new category of high-risk patients has emerged

Table 9.1 High-risk groups for thiamine deficiency and Wernicke's encephalopathy

Chronic alcoholism
Protracted vomiting (e.g. hyperemesis gravidarum)
Gastric resection and intestinal bypass
Starvation state (e.g. anorexia nervosa, radical diets)
Long-term intravenous alimentation
Chronic renal dialysis
Leukemia
Children with malignancy
Certain dietary restrictions (e.g. flour not enriched with
    thiamine)

Table 9.2 Causes of upbeat nystagmus

Wernicke's encephalopathy
Multiple sclerosis
Cerebellar degenerations
Focal lesions of vestibulocerebellum (tumor, stroke)
Midbrain lesions (tumor, stroke)
Brainstem encephalitis
Meningitis
Thalamic vascular malformation
Congenital
Organophosphate poisoning
Transient phenomenon in normal infants

in recent years with the increasing popularity of gastric surgery for obesity. Patients may be embarrassed about having had bariatric surgery and thus may not volunteer this aspect of their history, particularly during an evaluation for acute diplopia.

Ocular motor dysfunction is typically the earliest sign of Wernicke's encephalopathy. This may be as subtle as small-amplitude horizontal end-gaze nystagmus or slowing of saccades. Abduction weakness is common, sometimes manifest as just an esodeviation without a ductional deficit. Conjugate gaze palsies, which may be horizontal, vertical, or both, are present in almost half of cases. Upbeat nystagmus is also characteristic, due to disruption of the pathways connecting the anterior semicircular canal, cerebellum and brachia of the midbrain (see Table 9.2). About 30% of patients with Wernicke's encephalopathy have isolated or predominant mental status changes ranging from apathy, confusion and somnolence to delirium and frank coma. When the onset of symptoms is abrupt, Wernicke's encephalopathy may be mistaken for a stroke syndrome. This is particularly true in patients with sudden onset of a confusional state accompanied by esotropia. The presence of symmetric lesions in the paramedian thalamus in such cases may further add to the impression of a "top-of-the-basilar syndrome", i.e. occlusion of the posterior thalamoperforating arteries. In this clinical setting, an empiric trial of thiamine may have both diagnos-

tic and therapeutic value. Patients with Wernicke's encephalopathy typically experience rapid clearing of mental status and resolution of esotropia, whereas patients with stroke show no beneficial response.

The diagnosis of Wernicke's encephalopathy is made on clinical grounds. MRI findings, when present, can provide additional supportive evidence. Lesions are often symmetric with a predilection for the mamillary bodies, periventricular region of the third ventricle, medial thalamus, periaqueductal gray and midbrain tegmentum, seen best as hyperintensities on T2 and FLAIR sequences or as enhancement on post-contrast T1-weighted images (Figure 9.11). These abnormalities are quite specific for Wernicke's (93% specificity), but have relatively low sensitivity, present in only half of patients who are imaged within two weeks of symptom onset. Low serum erythrocyte transketolase activity confirms a state of thiamine deficiency but this test result may take days to obtain. Because the neurologic deficits of Wernicke's are reversible with prompt thiamine repletion, it is important to treat on suspicion, based on the clinical features as described above, rather than waiting for laboratory confirmation. Treatment usually starts with 100 mg of thiamine given intravenously or intramuscularly with glucose supplementation. Clinical manifestations often resolve within hours of thiamine repletion. Untreated, the condition can be life-threatening and associated with significant

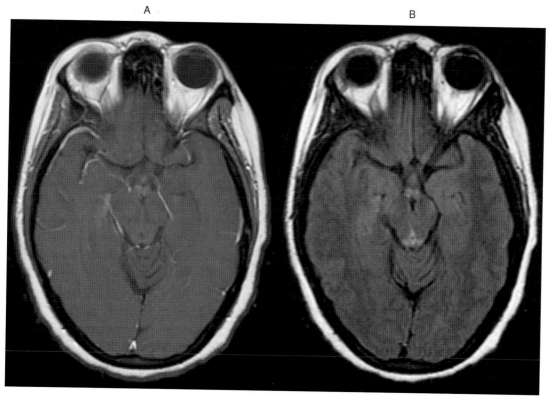

Figure 9.11 MRI of a different patient with Wernicke's encephalopathy. (A) Axial post-contrast T1-weighted image shows characteristic enhancement of the mamillary bodies. (B) Axial FLAIR image also demonstrates hyperintense signal in the dorsal midbrain and periaqueductal region. (Courtesy of Dr. Benjamin Kuzma.)

neurologic morbidity, including Korsakoff's amnesia as well as oculomotor and other brainstem deficits.

The clinical scenario: Conjugate gaze palsy and upbeat nystagmus

The look-alikes: Brainstem stroke vs. thiamine depletion (Wernicke's encephalopathy)

Tip: Eye movement abnormalities in Wernicke's encephalopathy are varied, and the classic clinical triad is frequently incomplete. Recognizing that the patient is at risk for thiamine deficiency is key to making the diagnosis.

Chronic progressive external ophthalmoplegia vs. progressive supranuclear palsy

Case: A 64-year-old retired plumber noted difficulty reading and trouble refocusing between distance and near. He was generally healthy but described progressive difficulty with balance for the preceding two years. Afferent visual function, pupillary examination and biomicroscopy were normal. Ocular motility testing revealed moderate limitation of horizontal eye movements and profound impairment of vertical gaze, especially downgaze, which was essentially absent. Saccades in all directions were markedly slowed. He had a small esophoria at distance and larger exophoria at near.

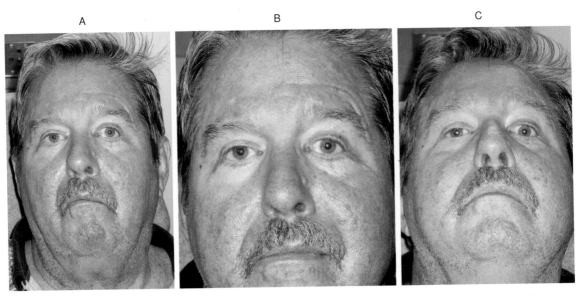

Figure 9.12 A 64-year-old man with PSP looking straight ahead (A) and attempting to look down on command (B). Notice that he cannot voluntarily move his eyes below primary position. When his head is tipped back quickly (C), downgaze is full, indicating the supranuclear basis for his ophthalmoplegia.

This combination of horizontal and vertical gaze limitation with slowed saccades could be due to either supranuclear gaze palsy or ocular myopathy. How can we distinguish these two mechanisms?

The status of reflex eye movements should differentiate these two disorders. The vestibulo-ocular reflex (Doll's head maneuver) is preserved, and even enhanced, in supranuclear gaze palsy, whereas in ocular myopathy (or any other disorder from the nucleus to the eye muscles), ocular excursions are no greater with reflex movements.

Although this patient had virtually no voluntary eye movement below midposition, when asked to fixate a target while his head was quickly tipped back, downgaze was full (Figure 9.12). The range of eye movements in other directions was similarly improved with reflex maneuvers. In performing this test, it was noted that there was some resistance to passive head movements. He also displayed a decreased blink rate and a general paucity of facial expression. Based on these clinical features,

a diagnosis of progressive supranuclear palsy (PSP) was made.

Discussion: Progressive supranuclear palsy is an idiopathic neurodegenerative disease characterized by parkinsonian features, subcortical dementia and supranuclear gaze palsy. The earliest manifestation is usually a non-specific gait disorder which usually precedes other symptoms by about two years. At this stage, it is not usually possible to make a definitive diagnosis. As the disease progresses, accurate diagnosis remains a challenge, reflected in the mean time from symptom onset to diagnosis of about four years. Typical neurologic features include increased axial tone, bradykinesia, dysarthria and dysphagia. Three clinical types of PSP have recently been distinguished. The most common is the classic syndrome described by Steele *et al.*, in which falls occur early in the course, tremor is absent, neurologic signs are symmetric and response to levodopa is poor. In one-third of patients, falls are delayed in onset and there is tremor, asymmetry, and a positive, though unfortunately transient, response to levodopa. Less commonly, gait apraxia is the initial and most prominent manifestation. With rare exceptions, ocular motor deficits are prominent in all three subtypes.

Most patients exhibit progressive loss of voluntary conjugate gaze, initially affecting vertical movements more than horizontal, and involving both pursuit and saccades. Prominent slowing of saccadic velocity is an invariable and sensitive sign. Pursuit is saccadic, consistent with cerebellar involvement, but nystagmus is not prominent due to loss of the fast (refixation) component. As the name indicates, the ophthalmoplegia in this disease is supranuclear so that reflex eye movements (Doll's head, Bell's phenomenon) are preserved as voluntary gaze is progressively lost. In more advanced cases, the Doll's head maneuver may be difficult to perform due to increased axial tone causing resistance to passive neck movement.

Vergence movements are also impaired, causing an exodeviation at distance and esodeviation at near. When diplopia occurs, it is due to this misalignment at varying distances rather than an imbalance in conjugate eye movements. Fixation is unstable, interrupted by frequent saccadic intrusions, termed *macro square wave jerks* based on their appearance on infrared oculography. The blink rate is decreased and some patients also experience blepharospasm and/or apraxia of eyelid opening. The constellation of eye movement abnormalities in this disease is so characteristic that the diagnosis can usually be made on clinical grounds.

There is no definitive test to confirm a diagnosis of PSP but clinical criteria established for research purposes have proved highly sensitive and specific. In addition, several characteristic MRI changes have been described. Atrophy of the dorsal midbrain is most prominent, sometimes causing an appearance on mid-sagittal sections termed the "hummingbird sign" in which thinning of the midbrain tegmentum mimics the tapered head and long, narrow beak of this bird (Figure 9.13). Additional changes that similarly reflect the predilection for certain areas of the brain in this disease include dilation of the posterior

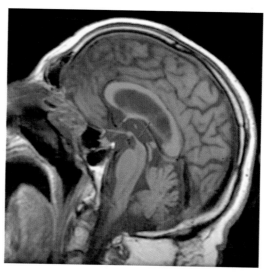

Figure 9.13 Mid-sagittal non-contrast T1-weighted MRI of a patient with PSP, showing the "hummingbird sign" due to thinning of the rostral end of the midbrain tegmentum (arrow). The tectal plate is thin and flat. (Photo courtesy of Dr. Benjamin Kuzma.)

third ventricle, atrophy of the anterior temporal lobes, iron deposition in the lateral putamen and wisps of high-T2 signal in the midbrain and pons due to gliosis. The role of functional imaging in the diagnosis of this disorder remains to be established.

Central cholinergic deficits are thought to be the basis for the postural instability, gait disturbance and cognitive impairment associated with PSP, however cholinergic replacement therapies have been generally ineffective. Management in patients with PSP remains symptomatic (see Chapter 12, Failure to provide symptomatic treatment). Unfortunately, the disease is relentlessly progressive and is usually fatal on average seven years after onset of symptoms.

Chronic progressive external ophthalmoplegia (CPEO) is similarly characterized by progressive, symmetric, bilateral loss of voluntary eye movements affecting horizontal and vertical gaze. The biochemical defect in this disorder consists of mutations or deletions of mitochondrial DNA that encode respiratory chain enzymes involved in the generation of adenosine triphosphate. Although CPEO is a widespread mitochondrial myopathy, symptoms are limited to eye muscles in most affected individuals. Bilateral ptosis usually develops during adolescence, followed by very slowly progressive limitation of eye movements over a lifetime. Eye muscles are usually affected so diffusely and symmetrically that patients do not experience diplopia. Some patients are completely asymptomatic and unaware of the ophthalmoplegia, their disease only uncovered during routine eye examination or evaluation for an unrelated condition. Examination shows limitation of eye movements with marked slowing of saccadic velocity, similar to the findings in PSP. In contrast to PSP, however, the range of eye movements in CPEO is *not* improved with reflex maneuvers. Skeletal muscle biopsy shows characteristic abnormal mitochondrial inclusions, termed *ragged red fibers* based on their appearance on trichrome stain, but the diagnosis can generally be made on clinical grounds. Treatment is supportive, including judicious ptosis surgery in selected cases. Periodic electrocardiograms should be obtained for early detection of cardiac conduction block that may occur in this syndrome.

The clinical scenario: Symmetric, bilateral ophthalmoplegia with slowed saccades

The look-alikes: PSP vs. CPEO

Tip: Reflex eye movements are preserved in PSP but are no better than voluntary eye movements in CPEO.

Orbital myositis vs. sixth nerve palsy

Case: A 28-year-old kindergarten teacher developed pain behind the right eye that was exacerbated by eye movement. The next day her pain was worse and she developed horizontal diplopia on right gaze. She was healthy and had no recent systemic symptoms or other focal deficits. Examination showed a small esotropia in primary position and incomplete

abduction of the right eye with brisk right lateral rectus saccades.

This patient's right abduction deficit suggested a sixth nerve palsy. What other mechanism might be responsible and what clinical features suggest this alternative cause?

While some intracranial causes of sixth nerve palsy are accompanied by ipsilateral pain, the presence of pain *with eye movement* indicates orbital pathology, usually due to inflammation. In addition, preservation of saccadic velocity in the presence of a ductional deficit suggests orbital restrictive disease. In contrast, sixth nerve weakness is accompanied by slowing of lateral rectus saccades. Closer inspection of this patient's right eye showed injection over the right medial rectus muscle, suggesting orbital pathology (Figure 9.14A). An orbital MRI revealed enlargement and enhancement of the right medial rectus muscle consistent with orbital myositis (Figure 9.14B) (see Chapter 2, Painful ptosis and diplopia). Ancillary testing for systemic inflammatory disorders was negative, and a diagnosis of idiopathic orbital myositis was made. She was treated with oral prednisone 80 mg/day and enjoyed prompt resolution of pain and progressive improvement of diplopia. Steroid treatment was tapered over three months then discontinued, and she remained well over the next two years of follow-up.

Discussion: In cases such as this one, it is helpful to start by first considering possible mechanisms for an abduction deficit, rather than assuming the presence of a cranial neuropathy. In addition to sixth nerve palsy, other potential mechanisms include a disease process involving the lateral rectus muscle (e.g. ischemia, inflammation or tumor), a transmission defect at the neuromuscular junction, and orbital restrictive disease. In this case, inflammatory swelling of the opposing medial rectus muscle has caused it to lose its normal elasticity, thus limiting abduction. Orbital inflammatory disease is almost always painful and is typically

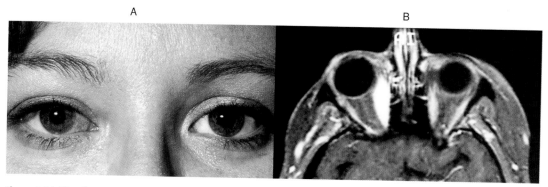

Figure 9.14 The above young woman with painful diplopia. (A) Note mild conjunctival injection medially in the right eye. (B) Axial post-contrast fat-suppressed T1-weighted MRI shows enlargement and intense enhancement of the right medial rectus muscle. There is also similar but milder enlargement of the left medial rectus muscle.

worse with eye movement. This historical feature is of great help in distinguishing these two mechanisms.

The clinical scenario: Isolated abduction deficit

The look-alikes: Sixth nerve palsy vs. orbital myositis

Tip: In a patient with acute diplopia, pain induced by eye movement indicates orbital inflammatory disease.

FURTHER READING

Optic neuritis vs. Leber's hereditary optic neuropathy

N. J. Newman, Hereditary optic neuropathies: from the mitochondria to the optic nerve. *Am J Ophthalmol*, **140** (2005), 517–23.

Optic Neuritis Study Group, The clinical profile of acute optic neuritis: experience of the Optic Neuritis Treatment Trial, *Arch Ophthalmol*, **109** (1991), 1673–8.

P. Riordan-Eva, M. D. Sanders, G. G. Govan *et al.*, The clinical features of Leber's hereditary optic neuropathy defined by the presence of a pathogenic mitochondrial DNA mutation. *Brain*, **118** (1995), 319–37.

Acute unilateral mydriasis

R. H. Kardon, O. Bergamin, Adie's pupil. In L. A. Levin, A. C. Arnold, eds., *Neuro-Ophthalmology: The Practical Guide.* New York: Thieme, 2005, pp. 325–39.

H. S. Thompson, Segmental palsy of the iris sphincter in Adie's syndrome. *Arch Ophthalmol*, **96** (1978), 1615–20.

Light near dissociation

D. M. Jacobson, R. A. Vierkant, Comparison of cholinergic supersensitivity in third nerve palsy and Adie's syndrome. *J Neuroophthalmol*, **18** (1998), 171–5.

R. H. Kardon, J. J. Corbett, H. S. Thompson, Segmental denervation and reinnervation of the iris sphincter as shown by infrared videographic transillumination. *Ophthalmology*, **105** (1998), 313–21.

H. S. Thompson, Light-near dissociation of the pupil. *Ophthalmologica*, **189** (1984), 21–3.

H. S. Thompson, R. H. Kardon, The Argyll Robertson pupil. *J Neuroophthalmol*, **26** (2006), 134–8.

Convergence spasm

R. V. P. Chan, J. D. Trobe, Spasm of accommodation associated with closed head trauma. *J Neuroophthalmol*, **22** (2002), 15–17.

L. R. Dagi, G. A. Chrousos, D. G. Cogan, Spasm of the near reflex associated with organic disease. *Am J Ophthalmol*, **103** (1987), 582–5.

N. J. Sarkies, M. D. Sanders, Convergence spasm. *Trans Ophthalmol Soc UK*, **104** (1985), 782–6.

Wernicke's encephalopathy

E. Antunez, R. Estruch, C. Cardenal *et al.*, Usefulness of CT and MR imaging in the diagnosis of acute Wernicke's encephalopathy. *AJR Am J Roentgenol*, **171** (1998), 1131–7.

C. Harper, Thiamine (vitamin B1) deficiency and associated brain damage is still common throughout the world and prevention is simple and safe! *Eur J Neurol*, **13** (2006), 1078–82.

K. Juhasz-Pocsine, S. A. Rudnicki, R. L. Archer, S. I. Harik, Neurologic complications of gastric bypass surgery for morbid obesity. *Neurol*, **68** (2007), 1843–50.

S. Singh, A. Kumar, Wernicke encephalopathy after obesity surgery. *Neurology*, **68** (2007), 807–11.

Progressive supranuclear palsy

N. Kato, K. Arai, T. Hattori, Study of the rostral midbrain atrophy in progressive supranuclear palsy. *J Neurol Sci*, **210** (2003), 57–60.

J. Schmiedel, S. Jackson, J. Schafer, H. Reichmann, Mitochondrial cytopathies. *J Neurol*, **250** (2003), 267–77.

J. C. Steele, J. C. Richardson, J. Olszewski, Progressive supranuclear palsy: a heterogeneous degeneration involving the brain stem, basal ganglia and cerebellum, with vertical gaze and pseudobulbar palsy, nuchal dystonia and dementia. *Arch Neurol*, **10** (1964), 333–59.

B. T. Troost, R. B. Daroff, The ocular motor defects in progressive supranuclear palsy. *Ann Neurol*, **2** (1977), 397–403.

Sixth nerve palsy vs. orbital myositis

G. E. Mannor, G. E. Rose, I. F. Moseley, J. E. Wright, Outcome of orbital myositis: clinical features associated with recurrence. *Ophthalmology*, **104** (1997), 409–14.

I. Mombaerts, L. Koornneef, Current status in the treatment of orbital myositis. *Ophthalmology*, **104** (1997), 402–8.

R. M. Siatkowski, H. Capo, S. F. Byrne, E. K. Gendron *et al.*, Clinical and echographic findings in idiopathic orbital myositis. *Am J Ophthalmol*, **118** (1994), 343–50.

10

Over-reliance on negative test results

In some cases, the correct diagnosis can be made based solely on information obtained from the history and physical examination. In other cases, we have a strong clinical suspicion regarding the diagnosis, which is then confirmed with specific ancillary testing. But, not uncommonly, the process is less direct and includes the formulation of a list of diagnostic possibilities, some of which are then eliminated based on additional studies. This activity is often referred to as "ruling out" this or that condition and common medical jargon reflects this process, so that the differential diagnosis is sometimes formulated as a list of "rule outs". As we embark on this process, it is important to have a critical awareness of the limitations of the tests that we use. When a test comes back with negative results, did we in fact "rule out" that disease?

Falsely negative test results may occur for several reasons. In rare instances, a mishap in laboratory handling, such as mixing up the specimens from two patients, produces an incorrect test result. In other cases, falsely negative results are related to technical problems in performing the test. An example of this is an obese patient with headaches and papilledema whose CSF pressure is spuriously low via lumbar puncture performed under fluoroscopy.

In some cases, false negative test results are related to the inherent limitations of the particular test. As revolutionary as MR scanning has been to the practice of neurology, there are certain diseases that just do not produce visible changes on neuro-imaging, and we look at a few such examples in this chapter. In other instances, a test may be quite sensitive when the disease process is generalized but is far less so when clinical manifestations are localized. This is often true for serum markers. For example, antineutrophilic cytoplasmic antibodies (ANCA) are positive in 97% of patients with systemic Wegener's granulomatosis but in only 40% of those with "limited" disease, e.g. isolated sino-orbital manifestations. Similarly, the angiotensin converting enzyme (ACE) level is less likely to be elevated in cases of sarcoidosis confined to the optic nerve than in cases with pulmonary involvement. In the case of giant cell arteritis, the multi-focal nature of the disease process leads to occasionally false-negative temporal artery biopsies.

The common thread in these cases is a discrepancy between the clinical findings and the results of ancillary testing. Increasing reliance on test results is a striking trend of modern medical practice. There is no question that it takes less time to order a test and read the results than it does to piece out the diagnosis from a detailed history and physical examination. But when the test results do not match the clinical diagnosis, it is important to have the confidence to set aside the report and pursue the diagnosis, and sometimes initiate treatment, based on one's clinical judgement. To this end, it is crucial to have a solid grounding in the clinical

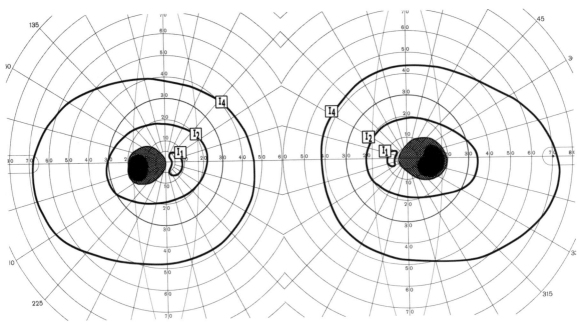

Figure 10.1 Goldmann visual field of a 59-year-old accountant shows bilateral ceco-central scotomas.

manifestations of these disorders and the limitations of the tests that we use to diagnose them.

Unexplained visual loss

Case: A 59-year-old accountant developed difficulty with near vision during her busy tax-preparation season. Along with blurring of vision in both eyes, she noticed that colors appeared less bright. There were no other focal deficits and no systemic symptoms. She was generally healthy and on no medications, had a normal diet, was a non-smoker and consumed occasional alcohol.

Examination showed best corrected visual acuity of 20/50 OD and 20/40 OS. She identified 7 of 15 Ishihara color plates in each eye and pupillary responses were normal. Goldmann perimetry revealed a relative ceco-central scotoma in each eye (Figure 10.1) and the fundus examination was completely normal. Laboratory testing showed a normal hemoglobin of 14 g/dL but elevated mean corpuscular volume (MCV) of 120 fL (normal 81–99). The

serum B12 level was 240 pg/mL (normal 220–1000). An MRI of brain and orbits with and without contrast was normal.

In the absence of any objective abnormalities, would you consider that this might be non-organic visual loss, perhaps due to job-related stress?

While this might be a consideration, the visual field pattern in this case (bilateral ceco-central scotomas) would be most unusual for functional visual loss. This particular visual field pattern usually indicates a disease process involving the papillomacular bundle. Specific forms of optic neuropathy that produce bilateral ceco-central scotomas include certain toxins, nutritional deficiencies, hereditary optic neuropathies and demyelinating disease (see Table 10.1). It is extremely unusual for this pattern of visual loss to be produced by a mass lesion; optic nerve or chiasmal compression can cause central loss but when it does there is almost always paracentral and/or peripheral field loss as well.

Table 10.1 Optic neuropathies that produce bilateral ceco-central scotomas

Toxins
   ethambutol
   isoniazide
   disulfiram
   chloramphenicol
   linezolide
   chemotherapy (cisplatin, vincristine, 5-FU)
Nutritional deficiency
   B-vitamins (B12, B6, B1)
   folate
Hereditary disorders
   Leber's hereditary optic neuropathy
   dominant optic atrophy
Demyelinating disease
   multiple sclerosis
   neuromyelitis optica

Visual loss due to nutritional deficiency was suspected based on her macrocytosis, however her serum B12 level was within the normal range. What would you like to do next?

There are other methods for investigating the possibility of B12 deficiency which might be helpful in this case. Because vitamin B12 is an important co-factor in the metabolism of homocysteine and methylmalonic acid, altered levels of these metabolites can be used as supportive evidence of a deficiency state. A comitant elevation of serum homocysteine (≥ 13 µmol/L) or methylmalonic acid (≥ 0.4 µmol/L) in the absence of renal failure, folate deficiency or insufficient level of B6 lends support to a diagnosis of B12 deficiency. A Schilling test is the standard method for demonstrating B12 malabsorption, but at many institutions this cumbersome test is no longer unavailable. Anti-parietal cell antibody assay is a useful test for the diagnosis of pernicious anemia although it is not helpful for identifying other mechanisms of B12 deficiency.

This patient's serum demonstrated a high titer of anti-parietal cell antibodies consistent with pernicious anemia. She was treated with 1000 micrograms of intramuscular hydroxycobalamin each week for one month followed by monthly injections. At her two-month follow-up visit, visual acuities had improved to 20/25 OU with normal color vision in each eye and the visual fields had returned to normal. She has been well on monthly maintenance B12 injections since.

Discussion: Vitamin B12 (cobalamin) deficiency is an important cause of optic neuropathy because visual loss is preventable and, to some extent, reversible with treatment. Important dietary sources of B12 are meat, liver, fish, cheese and eggs. The typical western diet contains 3–30 µg of B12 daily and hepatic reserves are sufficient for 5 to 10 years, thus symptoms of deficiency typically develop years after the causative event. Absorption of B12 requires gastric acid, pancreatic enzymes, intrinsic factor and intact mucosal cells in the ileum.

Those at risk for insufficient dietary intake of B12 are strict vegans, alcoholics, institutionalized patients and the elderly. The prevalence of cobalamin deficiency in the elderly population has been estimated at about 20%. A number of conditions can interfere with the normal absorption process of B12 and eventually lead to a deficiency state. These include gastrectomy, pernicious anemia, food-cobalamin malabsorption syndrome, pancreatectomy, and a variety of intestinal disorders (see Table 10.2). Food-cobalamin malabsorption syndrome is an increasingly recognized cause of B12 deficiency in patients with normal dietary intake and a normal Schilling test. The malabsorption stems from an inability to release cobalamin from ingested food so that it is unavailable for intrinsic factor-mediated absorption. The release of food cobalamin requires stomach pepsin and acid, so the main risk for this form of malabsorption is gastric dysfunction due to a number of underlying conditions (see Table 10.2).

The clinical sequelae of B12 deficiency can be divided into hematologic, neuropsychiatric and gastrointestinal manifestations. Hematologic changes consist of macrocytosis, hypersegmented neutrophils and anemia. Typical gastrointestinal

Table 10.2 Causes of vitamin B12 deficiency

Nutritional deficiency
   strict vegan diet
   alcoholism
   elderly
   institutionalized
Gastric disorders
   absence of intrinsic factors (pernicious anemia)
   gastroplasty/gastrectomy
   food-cobalamin malabsorption syndrome
      gastritis with achlorhydria
      gastric atrophy (Sjogren's syndrome, idiopathic)
      decreased acid (antacids, vagotomy)
      pancreatic disease (surgical, exocrine failure)
Small-bowel disorders
   intestinal surgery
   ileal disease (Crohn's, amyloid, lymphoma)
   infections (*Diphylloboturium latum*)

effects are indigestion and a smooth tongue (Hunter's glossitis). Neuropsychiatric changes are widespread, including combined sclerosis of the spinal cord, peripheral neuropathy, cognitive impairment, depression, parkinsonism and optic neuropathy. The visual loss of B12 deficiency is bilateral and symmetric, painless and gradually progressive. Loss of color vision, decreased acuity and central or ceco-central scotomas are characteristic. The optic discs may be normal or hyperemic acutely, pale and atrophic later.

Visual loss and other neurologic manifestations of B12 deficiency can occur well in advance of hematologic changes and therefore a CBC is not an adequate screening test for such vitamin deficiency. Furthermore, the official normal values provided by many laboratories indicate a rather broad range and occasional patients are symptomatically deficient even at levels that are technically within this normal range. This patient's visual loss was consistent with nutritional deficiency and she was therefore treated with parental hydroxycobalamin even though her B12 serum level was "officially" normal. Her positive response to treatment confirmed this as the mechanism of visual loss.

Diagnosis: Pernicious anemia with normal serum B12 level

Tip: The possibility of B12 deficiency should be entertained in patients with characteristic clinical features even in the presence of low-normal serum vitamin levels.

Twinkling after embolic stroke

Case: An 82-year-old woman was hospitalized for treatment of new-onset atrial fibrillation. At some point during her hospital course she developed difficulty seeing to the right side and a brain MRI revealed a left occipital infarct (Figure 10.2A). Soon after returning home she noticed continuous "sparkling and twinkling", along with mild photosensitivity. Over the next four months her sparkles persisted, especially in bright light, prompting neuro-ophthalmic consultation. On examination, visual acuity, pupillary responses and ophthalmoscopic appearance were normal. Goldmann perimetry showed a right homonymous superior quadrantanopic defect consistent with her left occipital infarct (Figure 10.2B).

Now we understand the basis of this patient's visual field defect. But what is causing her persistent photopsias?

This patient has suffered an embolic stroke secondary to atrial fibrillation. We would consider that the infarct may have produced cortical irritability, i.e. focal seizures, accounting for her positive visual symptoms. The continuous nature of her photopsias, however, would be extremely unusual, and an EEG was normal. Dilated examination of the fundi showed no retinal cause for her symptom.

It was noted that during her hospitalization the patient had been started on digoxin for persistent atrial fibrillation and had been on the same dose (0.25 mg/day) since discharge. The possibility of digitalis toxicity was considered, however her serum digoxin level was only 1.9 ng/ml (therapeutic

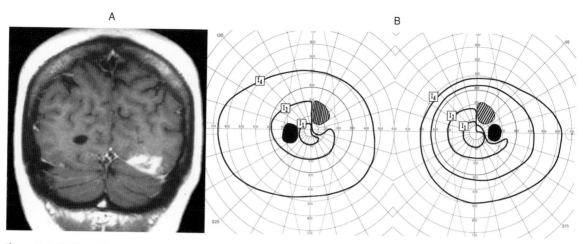

Figure 10.2 Radiographic and visual field findings in an 82-year-old woman with persistent "twinkling" after an embolic stroke. (A) Coronal post-contrast T1-weighted MRI shows abnormal left occipital cortical enhancement below the calcarine fissure, consistent with subacute infarction. (B) Goldmann perimetry reveals a corresponding congruous right homonymous superior quadrantic scotoma.

range 0.8–2.0 ng/ml). Despite her therapeutic level, this possibility was further pursued. Following discussion with her cardiologist, the digoxin dose was decreased to 0.125 mg per day and within one week her photopsias and light sensitivity completely resolved. She has since remained stable from a cardiovascular standpoint.

Discussion: Digitalis toxicity causes changes in many tissues, including the eye and brain. Visual dysfunction is probably due to its effects on photoreceptors, especially cones. While full-blown digitalis toxicity produces systemic effects including nausea, malaise, confusion and cardiac conduction abnormalities, visual manifestations may occur in the absence of other symptoms and signs. The classic description of digitalis toxicity emphasizes altered color vision, specifically the perception of a yellow-green tinge. In fact, there is a wide spectrum of visual disturbance associated with toxicity from cardiac glycosides, the most common of which is not yellow-green vision but white or "frosty" vision (see Table 10.3). Consistent with a predilection for causing cone dysfunction, visual symptoms from

Table 10.3 Visual symptoms of digitalis toxicity

Blurred or hazy vision
Alterations of color
   frosted or snowy vision
   xanthopsia
   less commonly red, blue or brown
Positive phenomena
   flashes, sparkles
   flickering, shimmering
   glare or dazzle
   scintillating scotoma

digitalis are most prominent in bright light and are often accompanied by positive visual phenomena and photosensitivity. Objective findings on examination include decreased acuity, abnormal color vision and central scotomas that are bilateral and symmetric.

Toxicity from cardiac glycosides may occur without a change in the dose or the addition of another medication. Furthermore, symptoms of toxicity may occur even with doses that are within the therapeutic range, as illustrated by this case. Abnormalities of color vision are demonstrable on the Farnsworth

Munsell 100-Hue test in 20% of patients with serum digitalis levels <1.5 ng/ml and in 50% of those with levels of 1.5–2.5 ng/ml.

The positive visual symptoms of digitalis toxicity are sometimes mistakenly attributed to other mechanisms such as posterior vitreous detachment, migraine, seizures and transient ischemic attacks. This diagnosis should be considered in any patient on cardiac glycosides who has unexplained visual loss or other afferent visual disturbance, particularly those with positive symptoms. The visual manifestations of digitalis are reversible upon stopping the medication or lowering the dose. Prompt recognition of this syndrome is also important because of the potentially life-threatening cardiac complications of digitalis toxicity.

Diagnosis: Digoxin toxicity with therapeutic levels

Tip: Visual manifestations of digitalis toxicity are varied and may occur even at serum levels that are within the therapeutic range.

Painless ptosis and diplopia

Case: A 66-year-old retired mathematics professor noted sudden painless drooping of his right upper eyelid and intermittent vertical diplopia. He found that tilting his head back alleviated his diplopia. Having chronic hypertension, a history of past tobacco use and a family history of cerebrovascular disease, he worried that he had suffered a small stroke and sought medical attention. His examination showed right upper lid ptosis with some variability and mildly limited supraduction of the right eye. Pupillary size and reactivity were normal. Neurologic examination revealed no other motor, sensory, cerebellar or cranial nerve dysfunction. Though the pattern of his motility deficit resembled a partial third nerve palsy, ocular myasthenia gravis was also considered. His physician was reluctant to perform a Tensilon (edrophonium chloride) test without electrocardiographic (ECG) monitoring due to the patient's vascular risk factors. Instead, an MRI and MRA were obtained to rule

out a compressive third nerve palsy. Neuro-imaging was normal. Acetylcholine receptor antibodies were normal and an electromyogram/nerve conduction study showed no decrement with repetitive nerve stimulation of limb and facial muscles. A presumptive diagnosis of brainstem stroke was given and an anti-platelet agent was prescribed.

Several months later, the patient was referred for worsening ptosis. A Tensilon test was now performed and was unequivocally positive (Figure 10.3). His diagnosis was changed to myasthenia gravis and additional evaluation and treatment were initiated accordingly.

Discussion: This case highlights the danger of relying on the acetylcholine receptor (AChR) antibody test for the diagnosis of myasthenia. In contrast to patients with generalized disease, who harbor autoantibodies in 90% or more of cases, fewer than half of patients with ocular myasthenia have a positive antibody test. The use of more recently identified autoantibodies only slightly increases the diagnostic yield. Blocking and modulating antibodies are positive in only 8% of patients in whom binding antibodies are negative, and MuSK antibodies are rarely positive in ocular myasthenia. While the sensitivity of myasthenic antibody testing is low, its appeal lies in its extremely high specificity. A positive test is essentially diagnostic.

Repetitive nerve stimulation studies of limb muscles are similarly normal in most patients with myasthenia limited to the ocular muscles. Single fiber electromyography (EMG) is more sensitive, however the test is not widely available and is highly examiner-dependent. Because of its high sensitivity, single fiber EMG testing sometimes yields results that are ambiguous or falsely positive.

There are several alternative methods for supporting a diagnosis of myasthenia. These include the ice test, the sleep test and pharmacologic testing with edrophonium chloride (Tensilon). Ptosis is a particularly good endpoint for these tests as it is sensitive and easy to observe and quantify. The *sleep test* is the simplest to perform. The patient lies quietly in a darkened room for 30–60 minutes with

A   B

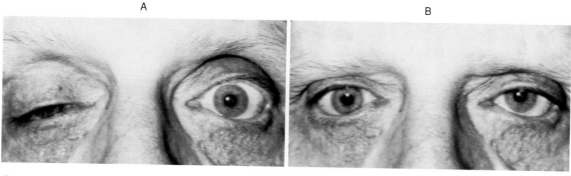

Figure 10.3 Positive Tensilon test in a 66-year-old gentleman with right upper lid ptosis and diplopia. (A) Baseline examination shows marked drooping of the right lid. There is also bilateral brow elevation due to excessive frontalis action and compensatory pseudo-retraction of the left upper lid. (B) Following intravenous injection of 6 mg of Tensilon, there is complete resolution of ptosis, consistent with myasthenia. Note also normalization of left upper lid and bilateral brow position.

eyes closed. A shorter version is the *rest test*, which requires only 2–5 minutes of non-forced eye closure. For the *ice test*, an ice pack is placed on the ptotic lid for 1–2 minutes. Some of the effectiveness of the ice test is related to the fact that the eyes are closed during the test, thus simulating the rest test. The ice test does appear to pick up a few additional cases by virtue of enhanced transmission at the neuromuscular junction at lower temperatures. Temporary improvement of ptosis after any of these maneuvers is considered a positive test. The sleep test and ice test have variable sensitivity and have not undergone rigorous controlled trials.

For the diagnosis of ocular myasthenia, the gold standard remains the Tensilon test. Some physicians are reluctant to perform Tensilon testing, either due to lack of familiarity with the mechanics of the test or because of concern regarding possible complications. In fact, serious complications of this test are rare. A physician survey based on 23 111 tests found serious side-effects in only 37 patients (0.16%). ECG monitoring is not routinely required for Tensilon testing in a healthy patient. A history of cardiac arrhythmia, use of atrio-ventricular (AV) nodal blockers and bronchospastic disease are considered relative contraindications to performing a Tensilon test, and in these settings it is appropriate to arrange for cardiac and respiratory monitoring.

Care must be taken in interpreting the results of Tensilon testing. In patients with diplopia, the preferred endpoint is always some form of ductional deficit (i.e. limitation of eye movement) rather than a tropia or phoria. In addition, the endpoint should not demonstrate marked baseline variability. A subjective judgement, such as the lids feeling less heavy or the eyes less strained, should never be used as the endpoint for the test. Falsely positive Tensilon tests are rare. If the clinical findings are consistent with myasthenia and the Tensilon test is positive, it is not necessary to embark on neuro-imaging to look for a different etiology. The take-away message here is not that every patient who is suspected of having myasthenia must have a Tensilon test. The pitfall is in believing that a diagnosis of myasthenia has been "ruled out" when the antibody test and/or EMG results are negative.

Diagnosis: Ocular myasthenia

Tip: Myasthenia gravis should be considered in the differential diagnosis of any painless, pupil-sparing ocular motor disorder. In contrast to its high sensitivity in the generalized form of the disease, antibody testing is positive in fewer than half of patients with ocular myasthenia.

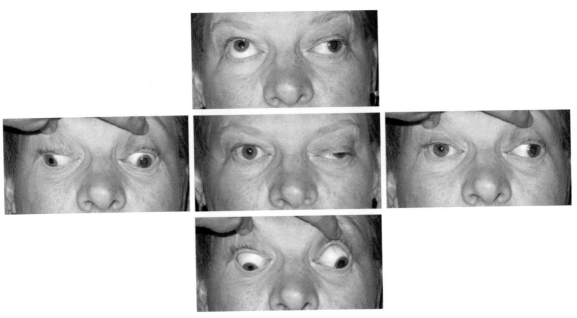

Figure 10.4 Ocular motility testing in a 52-year-old homemaker with a painful third nerve palsy. There is marked left upper lid ptosis and minimal movement of the left eye except for abduction. Notice also anisocoria, left pupil larger than right.

Headache and third nerve palsy

Case: A 52-year-old homemaker experienced sudden onset of a left-sided headache that increased in severity over two days. On the second day she noticed oblique diplopia followed by progressive drooping of her left upper lid. She had been previously healthy and specifically had no history of diabetes, hypertension or hypercholesterolemia. Examination showed a nearly complete left third nerve palsy with pupil involvement (Figure 10.4).

Which diagnostic possibilities should be addressed first?

The list of possible causes of an isolated acute third nerve palsy is lengthy (Table 10.4), but in this patient, some etiologies are more likely than others. The very acute onset speaks against a skull base tumor or infiltrative process such as nasopharyngeal carcinoma or chronic meningitis. An ischemic brainstem stroke can cause a third

Table 10.4 Causes of acute isolated and painful third nerve palsy

Compressive lesion
aneurysm
tumor
pituitary apoplexy
Ischemic
microvascular disease
vasculitis
carotid dissection
brainstem stroke
Inflammatory
sarcoidosis, tuberculosis, systemic lupus
idiopathic
Meningeal disease
infectious
neoplastic
Trauma

nerve palsy, but most cases are not accompanied by pain. The etiologies that should be addressed most urgently in this case are a posterior communicating artery aneurysm, pituitary apoplexy and

A

B

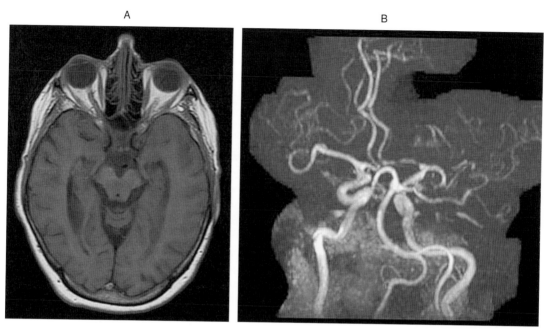

Figure 10.5 Neuro-imaging of the above patient. (A) Axial non-contrast T1-weighted MRI and (B) MRA maximum intensity projection reconstruction of the circle of Willis showed no cause for this patient's acute third nerve palsy.

carotid dissection, because in these conditions the outcome is most strongly influenced by the timeliness of treatment.

An MRI and MRA of the head were obtained and both were reportedly normal (Figure 10.5).

Based on her negative neuro-imaging, vasculopathic and inflammatory etiologies were considered. Serologic tests for systemic inflammatory diseases were all normal and the patient was treated with 60 mg per day of oral prednisone for a presumptive diagnosis of idiopathic inflammatory disease (see Chapter 6, Painful ophthalmoplegia). Her pain resolved in a few days but her extraocular muscle palsy and ptosis persisted. Eight weeks later, her examination was essentially unchanged and at that time she was referred for neuro-ophthalmic consultation.

What additional test should be obtained?

Although her pain improved with steroids, suggesting the possibility of Tolosa Hunt syndrome,

her motility did not show the expected recovery, effectively eliminating this diagnosis. Is her clinical course at this point consistent with a vasculopathic third nerve palsy? Failure to show some degree of recovery eight weeks after onset speaks strongly against an ischemic cranial nerve palsy (see Chapter 11, Acute isolated sixth nerve palsy). At this point no cause for this patient's third nerve palsy has been found, despite a variety of ancillary tests, and we must therefore reconsider the diagnoses that have previously been excluded. Of these possibilities, the most threatening is a *cerebral aneurysm* and it is important to ask if this diagnosis has been fully excluded. The essence of this case is whether a negative MRA truly "rules out" an aneurysm. An acute, painful, pupil-involving third nerve palsy in a young or middle-aged adult with no vascular risk factors is so strongly suggestive of a posterior communicating artery aneurysm that we must go the extra mile to exclude it. This patient therefore had a conventional carotid arteriogram that did reveal an aneurysm at the junction of the

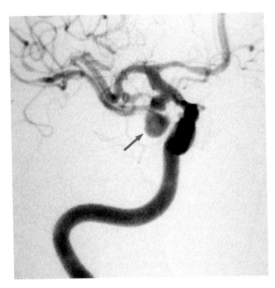

Figure 10.6 Left internal carotid arteriogram (catheter study) of the same patient. A bilobed saccular aneurysm projects inferiorly from the posterior communicating artery (arrow). In retrospect, the more proximal lobe of the aneurysm is in fact present on the MRA reconstruction (Figure 10.5).

left internal carotid and posterior communicating arteries (Figure 10.6). The source films from the original MRA were subsequently reviewed by the neuroradiologist who had performed the catheter angiogram and the aneurysm was identifiable. The patient underwent clipping of her aneurysm and her third nerve palsy showed partial resolution over the next six months.

Discussion: As the sensitivity of non-invasive imaging improves, the need for conventional arteriography decreases. At this point, magnetic resonance angiography (MRA) and computed tomography angiography (CTA) are extremely sensitive for the detection of cerebral aneurysms, but have not yet achieved 100% accuracy. A recent study comparing MRA techniques to catheter angiography in patients with third nerve palsy due to an unruptured posterior communicating artery aneurysm found a sensitivity of 92% using reformatted images and 98% using source image

analysis. Studies using CTA have reported a similarly high sensitivity for the detection of symptomatic aneurysms. The sensitivity of these techniques depends in part on the size of the aneurysm. The ability of MRA or CTA to detect an aneurysm approaches 100% for aneurysms larger then 5 mm; however, the risk of aneurysmal rupture for aneurysms smaller than 5 mm can approach 10%.

In addition, and perhaps more importantly, clinicians must be cautious in applying data from published series to their own practice. The level of non-invasive technology available at a particular community hospital may not be equivalent to that of a tertiary care center. This disparity is due to several factors, including differences in magnet strength and other aspects of instrumentation, imaging acquisition and processing, and the expertise of the person who interprets the images.

Although MRA and CTA are not quite as sensitive as catheter angiography, not all negative studies should be followed by an angiogram. As in all such medical decisions, the risks of each study must be weighed against its benefits. In patients with a low likelihood of harboring an aneurysm, and particularly in those who also have a relatively high risk for complications from an arteriogram, an MRA or CTA is the more appropriate study. Patients who would be considered to have a relatively low risk of aneurysm would include those who are being screened for an aneurysm because of polycystic kidney disease or because of a family member with an aneurysm. Those who have a similarly low risk of aneurysm and, additionally, a high risk of complications from invasive angiography, are older patients with vascular risk factors who develop an acute pupil-sparing but partial third nerve palsy or a complete palsy with slight pupil involvement. In such cases, a negative MRA or CTA is usually sufficient, with the caveat that the patient be monitored for possible development of pupillary involvement over the next 7 to 10 days. In patients with an otherwise complete but pupil-sparing, isolated third nerve palsy with vascular risk factors, no imaging is needed. These patients can be followed expectantly, watching for spontaneous recovery over the next 6 to 12 weeks.

In summary, neither MRA nor CTA fully replaces conventional arteriography in the investigation of a possible cerebral aneurysm. Non-invasive angiography may be the first choice in many situations because of its availability and excellent safety profile, but it is not necessarily the last choice. The potential consequences of missing an aneurysm are grave. The mortality rate following a ruptured intracerebral aneurysm ranges from 25 to 50% and, of the survivors, another 50% remain severely neurologically disabled.

Diagnosis: Aneurysmal third nerve palsy

Tip: If the clinical findings strongly suggest an aneurysm, a conventional arteriogram should either be obtained initially or, if non-invasive tests are performed first and are unrevealing, as a follow-up study.

Truly negative neuro-imaging

There are a number of potential pitfalls in the area of radiographic testing. In Chapter 4 (Radiographic errors) we looked at some examples of scans in which an abnormality was present but overlooked. In this section we consider a different type of error: cases in which the scan is truly normal, even upon retrospective review, because the disease process is simply not visible on the imaging study. This may occur because imaging is obtained too early in the disease process, for example an ischemic event that is not apparent on CT scan for the first 24 hours. In other cases, the disease process is a metabolic one that does not produce changes on routine imaging studies, for example parkinsonian syndromes and certain dementias. In yet other instances, the disease process is simply below the resolving power of the scanner. In cases such as these, the clinical findings assume even greater importance, forcing us to rely on "old-fashioned" clinical diagnosis, as in the pre-MRI era.

Brainstem syndrome with negative scan

Case: A 35-year-old, previously healthy construction worker experienced new onset of painless double vision and difficulty looking to the side. Afferent visual function was normal. Motility testing showed complete loss of left gaze in both eyes and loss of adduction in the left eye (Figure 10.7). Abducting saccades in the right eye were brisk but all other horizontal saccades were profoundly slowed. There was abduction nystagmus in the right eye. General neurologic testing showed a mild left peripheral facial palsy and was otherwise normal.

Can you localize this patient's lesion?

This patient has a classic *"one-and-a-half" syndrome* consisting of a left conjugate gaze palsy with left internuclear ophthalmoplegia (INO), indicating a lesion of the left paramedian pons. These ocular motor findings are due to involvement of the paramedian pontine reticular formation (PPRF) or sixth nerve nucleus, plus interruption of the adjacent medial longitudinal fasciculus on that side. This constellation of clinical findings is exquisitely localizing (Figure 10.8). Frequent associated deficits include skew deviation, gaze-evoked upbeat nystagmus with impaired vertical pursuit, and ipsilateral facial palsy.

What is the most likely etiology in this patient and how would you proceed with the evaluation?

Disorders that cause the "one-and-a-half syndrome" are the same as those that produce INO, most commonly demyelinating disease in younger individuals and stroke in older patients. More unusual etiologies include brainstem hemorrhage, tumor, cavernous hemangioma, trauma and inflammation. This patient had a brain MRI with and without contrast which showed no abnormality in the pons at the expected site of damage, but did show two clinically asymptomatic, periventricular hemispheric white matter lesions (Figure 10.9). A

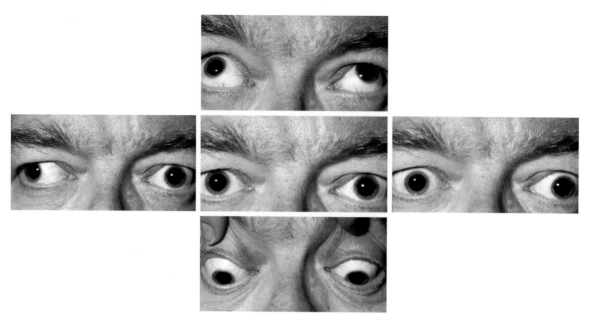

Figure 10.7 Ocular motility in the above 35-year-old construction worker with acute painless diplopia. Vertical gaze is normal but there is complete loss of horizontal movements in the left eye and loss of adduction in the right eye. (The pupils are pharmacologically dilated.)

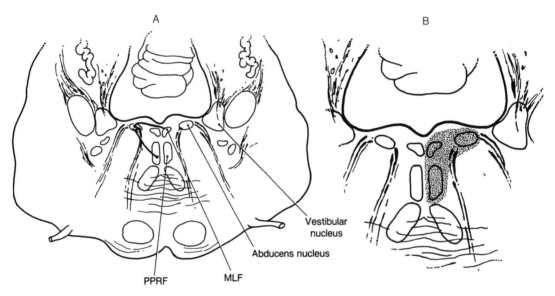

Figure 10.8 Location of lesion producing the one-and-a-half syndrome. (A) The important structures involved in the production of horizontal gaze. MLF: medial longitudinal fasciculus, PPRF: paramedian pontine reticular formation. Neurons project from the PPRF to the abducens nucleus which contains both motor neurons whose axons represent the abducens nerve and internuclear neurons whose axons ascend in the contralateral MLF. (B) The areas that may be involved in a one-and-a-half syndrome (shaded). Involvement of either the abducens nucleus or the PPRF can cause the horizontal gaze palsy. Damage to the ipsilateral medial longitudinal fasciculus produces the internuclear ophthalmoplegia. (From *Walsh and Hoyt's Clinical Neuro-Ophthalmology*, 6th edn. N. R. Miller, N. J. Newman, V. Biousse, J. B. Kerrison, eds. Philadelphia: Lippincott Williams and Wilkins, 2005, Vol. 1, Chapter 19, p. 924, with permission.)

A   B

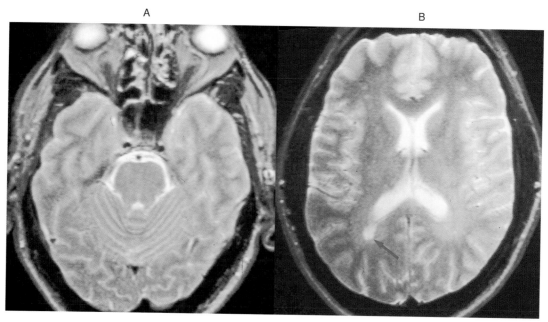

Figure 10.9 MRI of the above patient with an acute, left one-and-a-half syndrome. (A) Axial FLAIR image through the pons shows no abnormality, but a higher section (B) shows a hyperintense white matter lesion adjacent to the occipital horn of the right lateral ventricle (arrow). A second lesion was seen adjacent to the left anterior horn on a higher image (not shown).

subsequent lumbar puncture revealed an elevated IgG index, confirming the clinical diagnosis of an acute demyelinating event.

Discussion: Despite continued advances in neuro-imaging, some pathologic processes, even when focal, elude radiographic detection. In some cases, the disease process does not produce changes on CT or MRI until late in the course. In other cases, such as this one, the focal pathologic process is simply below the resolving power of the scan. This patient's MRI was performed on a 1.5 Tesla machine and included 5 mm sections using standard T1-weighted images with contrast, and T2-weighted images as well as diffusion-weighted and fluid-attenuated inversion recovery (FLAIR) sequences. FLAIR images are the most sensitive sequence for detecting demyelinating disease, but did not detect the responsible lesion in this case. Early ischemic lesions are best seen on diffusion-weighted images

(DWI) but this sequence has the disadvantage of relatively low spatial resolution. Thus, patients with comparable brainstem events due to lacunar infarction may have similarly unrevealing scans. The lesion responsible for this patient's clinically isolated brainstem syndrome was not visible on any of these MRI sequences but two larger, though asymptomatic, periventricular lesions were seen on FLAIR images. The combination of clinical and radiographic findings in this case led to the diagnosis of an isolated demyelinating event.

Diagnosis: One-and-a-half syndrome secondary to a clinically isolated demyelinating event

Tip: Some lesions are simply below the resolving power of current MR scans. In cases with exquisitely localizing neurologic deficits, the clinical information trumps the scan.

Homonymous hemianopia with negative neuro-imaging

Case: A 60-year-old farmer developed progressive difficulty seeing to the left. This was initially an isolated symptom, with no other focal deficits, alteration of mental status or systemic symptoms. Two weeks later he developed, in addition, some clumsiness and mild confusion. Ophthalmic examination four weeks after onset showed a fairly dense left homonymous hemianopia with otherwise normal findings. A stroke or tumor of the right occipital lobe was suspected, but an MR scan was normal.

What disease processes would you consider here?

The list of diseases that can produce focal occipital dysfunction without accompanying MRI changes is a short one: non-ketotic hyperglycemia, Alzheimer's disease, Creutzfeldt–Jakob disease, complicated migraine, hypoxic-ischemic encephalopathy and occipital seizures (ictal or post-ictal). This patient's blood glucose and electrolytes were normal and he had no personal or family history of migraine. His course was thought to be too rapid for Alzheimer's disease. A lumbar puncture was positive for the 14-3-3 protein and he received a diagnosis of Creutzfeldt–Jakob disease. He was given supportive care and over the next several weeks he exhibited further cognitive decline with new onset of frequent myoclonic jerks. He passed away at home eight weeks after onset of his symptoms.

Discussion: Creutzfeldt–Jakob disease (CJD) is one of several spongiform encephalopathies caused by a transmissible pathogenic form of the prion protein, a normal constituent of cell membranes. Prion diseases affect animals and humans, have a long incubation period before onset of neurologic deterioration and are invariably fatal. In animals, the pathogenic prion is transmitted during direct contact with an infected animal or by consumption of infected feed. Animal prion diseases include scrapie, bovine spongiform encephalopathy (so-called "mad cow disease") and transmissible mink encephalopathy.

Human prion disease can be divided into familial forms (familial CJD, Gerstmann–Straussler–Scheinker disease and fatal familial insomnia), non-familial CJD (sporadic, variant and iatrogenic types) and kuru. Only 10–15% of cases in humans are familial. In the majority of human cases the mode of transmission is unknown. Occasional cases result from iatrogenic infection, occurring in recipients of dural grafts, corneal transplants and growth hormone extract from cadaver pituitary glands. In a remote region of New Guinea, a prion disease known as *kuru* was found to be transmitted by the ancient practice of ritual cannibalism during bereavement ceremonies. Once reaching epidemic proportions several decades ago, kuru has nearly disappeared since the suppression of cannibalism. In the mid 1990s a clustering of cases in Great Britain was linked to an outbreak of bovine spongiform encephalopathy, although the exact route of transmission was unclear. These patients were clinically and histopathologically distinct from the more common sporadic form of CJD. Termed *variant CJD* (vCJD), these patients were younger (mean age 29 years), had a more protracted period of psychiatric symptoms before onset of dementia and death, and did not show the typical electroencephalography (EEG) and MRI changes of sporadic CJD.

Sporadic CJD is the most common form of human prion disease. It has no geographic or gender preference and the average age at onset is 60 years. Its mode of transmission is unknown. Neurologic manifestations of sporadic CJD are varied, most commonly taking the form of rapidly progressive dementia with myoclonic jerks. In some patients, the disease presents primarily as a progressive cerebellar syndrome; in others amyotrophy is prominent. In one particular form, the brunt of the disease process affects the posterior cerebral hemispheres, causing homonymous defects, cortical blindness and a variety of higher cortical visual deficits. This form is referred to as the *Heidenhain variant* and, for reasons that are unclear, it has a more rapidly progressive course than other forms. As in other forms of prion disease, there is no known treatment and death is inevitable.

The diagnosis of sporadic CJD can be suspected on clinical grounds and is confirmed with brain biopsy, which shows a characteristic triad of spongiform change, neuronal loss and gliosis. Amyloid plaques are found in 10% of cases and immunocytochemical staining for the protease-resistant prion protein associated with the disease is uniformly present. Characteristic EEG changes consist of diffuse slowing with periodic high-amplitude biphasic or tri-phasic discharges. CSF markers such as the 14-3-3 protein, neuron-specific enolase and total Tau are also helpful in diagnosis, but are not uniformly present and may also be present in other neurologic conditions. MRI is more reliable than CSF markers in the diagnosis of CJD. Characteristic patterns of hyperintense signal abnormalities involving the cerebral cortex and basal ganglia have been described and have a greater than 90% specificity for CJD. In sporadic CJD, the caudate nucleus and putamen are typically involved, whereas variant CJD affects the pulvinar of the thalamus. Initially described on T2-weighted images, abnormal signal changes are better detected using proton density, FLAIR or diffusion-weighted MRI sequences. Although more than half of patients with CJD eventually show characteristic MRI abnormalities, early in the course of the disease routine MRI sequences are often normal.

Diagnosis: Creutzfeldt–Jakob disease (Heidenhain variant).

Non-dominant parietal lobe syndrome with negative neuro-imaging

Case: A 61-year-old chemistry professor experienced slowly progressive visual difficulty over a four-year period. Specifically, she described a tendency to lose her place on the page when reading, lecturing or playing music. She sometimes misreached for objects and would often veer to the right when driving. A general ophthalmic examina-

tion was normal except for a left homonymous inferior quadrantanopic defect (Figure 10.10). Neurologic testing showed an alert and attentive woman with fluent speech and good repetition. She was able to recall three objects at five minutes and could read fluently. She exhibited marked impairment, however, on tests of spatial organization, including difficulty copying figures, matching shapes, and filling in the numbers on a clock, along with evidence of left-sided neglect (Figure 10.11). Thyroid function tests, a serum B12 level, FTA and metabolic panel were all normal as was a brain MRI with contrast.

Can you localize this patient's problem?

This patient displays a deficit of spatial organization, manifest as constructional apraxia and left-sided neglect, pointing to dysfunction involving the right (non-dominant) parietal lobe. Her visual field defect is also consistent with this localization. Based on her slowly progressive course and unrevealing work-up, a presumptive diagnosis of Alzheimer's disease was made. Over the next three years she experienced further difficulty with cognitive tasks including trouble with calculations and memory deficits and was forced to retire from teaching because of these symptoms. A positron emission tomography (PET) scan performed five years after onset of symptoms showed hypometabolism in the posterior cerebral hemispheres, consistent with Alzheimer's disease (Figure 10.12).

Discussion: Alzheimer's disease is the most frequent dementing disorder affecting the elderly. It is characterized by insidious onset of progressive cognitive decline and by its unique pathology. While generally thought of as a diffuse dementing process, the hallmark neuropathologic findings in Alzheimer's disease (neuritic plaques and neurofibrillary tangles) are not evenly distributed in the cortex but are rather concentrated in areas of greater neuronal vulnerability. Functional imaging studies have corroborated this regional susceptibility, demonstrating hypometabolism primarily in the

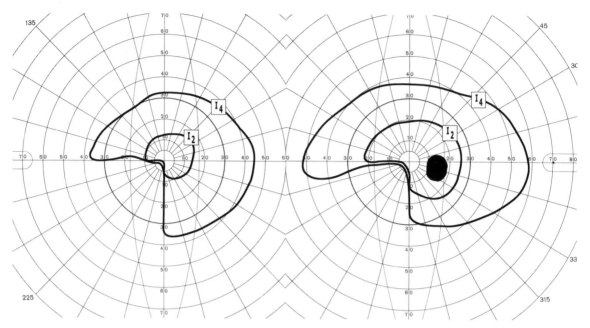

Figure 10.10 Goldmann perimetry in a 61-year-old chemistry professor shows a mildly incongruous left inferior quadrantanopia.

posterior parietal lobes and adjacent temporal and occipital cortex.

In keeping with the neuropathologic findings, the clinical features, especially in the early stage of disease, often manifest as selective rather than global cognitive dysfunction, such as word-finding difficulty or problems with calculations. Patients in whom the brunt of the disease affects the right posterior parietal lobe typically present with visual symptoms related to spatial disorganization, as in the above case, sometimes referred to as the *"visual variant of Alzheimer's disease"*. In the later stages of the disease, when both posterior hemispheres are involved, patients have even more profound visual difficulty, including inability to attend to more than one visual stimulus at a time, termed *simultanagnosia*. When accompanied by *"optic ataxia"* (difficulty pointing to a target) and *"psychic paralysis of gaze"* (difficulty directing the eyes toward an object of interest) this is termed Balint's syndrome and indicates bilateral damage to the posterior visual

association areas. Recognition of these visual presentations of Alzheimer's disease is particularly relevant to eye care providers who are often the first to be consulted for these patients' initial symptoms. The diagnosis in such cases may be challenging, as cognitive function is otherwise unimpaired and routine neuro-imaging is unrevealing. Functional imaging studies may be particularly helpful in this setting.

In addition to these higher cortical deficits, there are other mechanisms which may affect vision in patients with Alzheimer's disease. There is histopathologic evidence of progressive retinal ganglion cell loss, particularly affecting M-cell pathways, which are thought to be involved in global interpretation of spatial organization based on motion and depth discrimination. In addition, patients with Alzheimer's disease display a variety of ocular motility abnormalities including fixational instability, prolonged saccadic latency, poor tracking, and loss of saccadic velocity

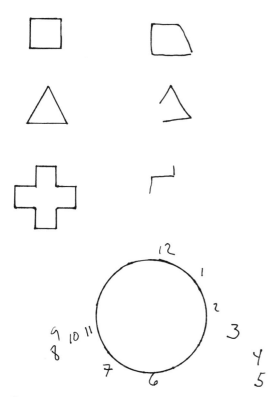

Figure 10.11 Constructional testing in the above patient with symptoms of spatial disorganization. The drawings (top) on the right represent the patient's efforts to copy the figures on the left. Below, the patient was asked to fill in the numbers as they would appear on a clock.

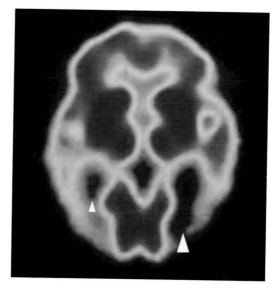

Figure 10.12 Axial PET scan of the above patient shows hypometabolism in the parietal-occipital regions (arrowheads), which is more prominent on the right side (larger arrowhead). Areas with higher metabolic activity appear red, those with lowest activity are dark blue and intermediate areas are green to yellow.

and accuracy, which may further impair visual function.

In this case and the preceding one, the leading edge of a dementing illness was a homonymous hemianopia. The underlying disease process in the first patient was Creutzfeld–Jacob disease and, in this patient, Alzheimer's disease. In each case, the pathologic process was not seen on MRI, not because the lesion was too small or because it was overlooked, but because these particular degenerative processes do not generally produce visible changes on routine neuro-imaging studies. In the second patient, the pathology was eventually demonstrated with functional imaging. Although these two disorders share some common features,

the time course of each is sufficiently different to enable differentiation in most cases. Non-ketotic hyperglycemia, migraine, hypoxic encephalopathy and post-ictal states can similarly produce a homonymous hemianopia with negative neuro-imaging, but the acute nature of those syndromes is distinctive and in such cases the main differential is an ischemic stroke (Table 10.5).

Table 10.5 Conditions producing cortical visual loss with negative MRI

Alzheimer's disease
Creutzfeldt–Jakob disease
Non-ketotic hyperglycemia
Migraine
Seizures (ictal and post-ictal)
Hypoxic-ischemic encephalopathy

Diagnosis: Visual variant of Alzheimer's disease

Tip: Certain dementing disorders may produce *focal* signs and symptoms along with (and sometimes preceding) more widespread cerebral dysfunction. Despite striking clinical deficits, MRI correlates may be absent in such cases.

Progressive third nerve palsy

Case: A 53-year-old, previously healthy farmer experienced left upper lid ptosis and diplopia associated with a dull ipsilateral headache. He noted decreased movement of the left eye, which progressively worsened over the next three months. His examination revealed an isolated, partial left third nerve palsy without pupillary involvement (Figure 10.13).

An MR scan with contrast was entirely normal, including thin coronal sections through the region of the cavernous sinus and superior orbital fissure. A cerebral arteriogram, lumbar puncture with cytologic examination and a variety of serologic tests for inflammatory diseases were also unrevealing. His fasting blood glucose was normal but the two-hour post-prandial level was mildly elevated. A diagnosis of vasculopathic (ischemic) cranial nerve palsy was considered but was felt to be incompatible with his slowly progressive three-month course. This time course and his persistent pain were strongly suggestive of an inflammatory or neoplastic process, but high-quality neuro-imaging was negative.

What other investigations might be helpful?

Otolaryngology (ENT) consultation was subsequently obtained. Direct and mirror examination of the nasopharynx was unremarkable but several biopsy specimens were obtained, two of which were positive for malignancy. Histopathologic examination revealed a cylindroma, a form of nasopharyngeal carcinoma. There was no evidence of metastatic disease and he was treated with 6000 cGy of external beam radiation.

Discussion: This case again highlights the differential diagnosis for an isolated painful third nerve palsy. A malignant skull base tumor was eventually

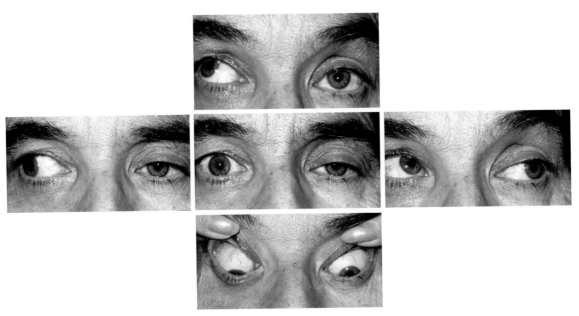

Figure 10.13 Motility examination in a 53-year-old farmer with a partial left third nerve palsy of three months' duration. There is moderate left upper lid ptosis and limitation of elevation of the left eye with milder loss of adduction and depression.

diagnosed but, even in retrospect, there was no evidence of the tumor on his scan. Nasopharyngeal carcinoma is notorious for infiltrating along the skull base and picking off cranial nerves while remaining below the radar screen on radiographic testing.

Another setting in which repeated neuro-imaging may be negative despite progressive cranial nerve palsy is the patient who develops a sixth nerve palsy one to two years after excision and radiation treatment of a head/neck tumor. In the face of negative diagnostic studies, radiation damage is often considered. Unlike the afferent visual pathways, however, the ocular motor nerves are relatively resistant to radiation necrosis. Sadly, these patients almost invariably turn out to have recurrent tumor at the skull base, despite scans that purportedly "ruled out" this process. Patients with peri-neural spread of squamous cell carcinoma represent a similar challenge. These patients typically develop pain and numbness in the area of a previously excised tumor, then progress to involvement of the seventh nerve on that side, often with other cranial neuropathies appearing in the course of the disease. Even high-quality neuro-imaging in these patients can be surprisingly normal, despite involvement of multiple cranial nerves. Ultra-thin sections with specialized views of the skull base and foramina can demonstrate subtle changes in many cases. When bony erosion is present in such cases, it is best demonstrated on CT of the skull base using thin-section bone windows.

Diagnosis: Third nerve palsy secondary to nasopharyngeal carcinoma

Tip: ENT evaluation should be included in the evaluation of any patient with an unexplained, progressive and painful ophthalmoplegia. Soft tissue biopsy may be diagnostic, even in the absence of visible changes on radiographic studies or direct nasopharyngeal examination.

Upgaze palsy

Case: A 14-year-old girl presented with recent onset of headaches and blurred vision. A ventriculoperito-

neal shunt had been placed at one month of age for hydrocephalus associated with a Chiari Type II malformation. Her shunt was revised at age 3 years, and again at age 7, and then at age 10 a new shunt was placed in the left lateral ventricle. She was otherwise healthy and there was no history of recent illness or trauma. Examination showed an alert and attentive teenager. Pupils were 7 mm in room light and sluggishly reactive to a bright light but more responsive to near effort. Upward gaze was full in both eyes when following a slowly moving target but was incomplete when tested with saccades. Attempts to look up quickly precipitated brief, repetitive movements of both eyes that were difficult to characterize in terms of direction. There was no papilledema and the examination was otherwise normal. A CT scan showed the shunt to be in its expected place in the frontal horn of the left lateral ventricle. The scan showed a mildly enlarged occipital horn on the right side which was unchanged from her previous scans. There was no generalized ventriculomegaly. A subsequent MRI also showed no acute changes (Figure 10.14).

What do you make of this patient's negative neuro-imaging in light of her clinical presentation?

This patient presented with the classic findings of a *dorsal midbrain syndrome,* also termed *Parinaud's syndrome* or the *syndrome of the superior colliculus.* In patients with an intraventricular shunt, the appearance of signs or symptoms of dorsal midbrain dysfunction is an early clinical signal of shunt malfunction. Her scans, however, did not show ventricular dilation as expected. Despite her negative imaging, shunt malfunction was strongly suspected on clinical grounds and she was therefore taken to surgery for shunt exploration. The shunt was found to be obstructed at the proximal end. Following revision, her headaches resolved and eye findings improved although she was left with mild impairment of upgaze.

Discussion: The dorsal midbrain syndrome typically includes upgaze palsy, retraction-convergence

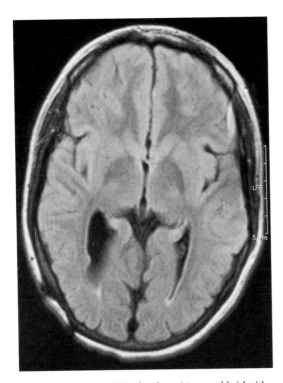

Figure 10.14 Brain MRI in the above 14-year-old girl with Chiari II malformation and recent onset of headaches. Axial FLAIR image shows mild enlargement of the right occipital horn, unchanged from its appearance on previous scans but there is no generalized ventriculomegaly and no subependymal resorption of fluid.

nystagmus, lid retraction (Collier's sign) and poorly reactive pupils with light-near dissociation (see Chapter 9, Chronic tonic pupils vs. Argyll Robertson pupils), although not all findings are uniformly present. Retraction-convergence nystagmus is distinctive but often difficult to characterize on examination, especially if the examiner is unfamiliar with it. The nystagmus is due to repeated, synchronous co-firing of third nerve muscles. The upward and downward components cancel out in terms of direction, resulting in globe retraction that is best detected by observing the patient's eyes from the side, i.e. profile view. Bilateral medial rectus contractions are unopposed and produce con-

vergent movements along with the retraction. In some cases the convergence component is absent. These abnormal eye movements are precipitated by attempts at upward saccades and can be elicited by asking the patient to quickly look up at a target. They are even more evident with a downward-moving optokinetic nystagmus (OKN) tape, which normally elicits repeated upward saccades. Retraction-convergence nystagmus can be quite pronounced acutely and usually diminishes over time.

The dorsal midbrain syndrome is most often caused by a mass lesion, either by direct compression from a pineal region tumor or due to an intrinsic tectal tumor. In cases of hydrocephalus without such a tumor, a dilated third ventricle can act as a mass lesion, compressing the dorsal midbrain and causing similar symptoms. Less commonly, this syndrome is caused by inflammation, ischemia, hemorrhage or demyelination in this region. In patients with a ventriculoperitoneal shunt, the development of the dorsal midbrain syndrome usually signifies shunt malfunction and radiographic studies typically show ventricular enlargement.

Occasionally, however, the ventricles in such patients are not enlarged, giving the mistaken impression that the shunt is working properly. The mechanism of neurologic dysfunction in such cases is thought to involve an increase in water in the periaqueductal tissue due to increased pressure within the aqueduct. This in turn causes decreased cerebral blood flow in the periventricular white matter. This sequence of events is particularly likely in children who have undergone shunting and is probably due to decreased compliance of the ventricle walls as a result of subependymal gliosis. In some of these cases, the MR scan shows periventricular hyperintensity, most prominent on T2-weighted and FLAIR sequences, indicating subependymal resorption of fluid (Figure 10.15B), but such changes are not uniformly present. In some cases the ventricles are unusually small, termed "slit ventricle syndrome", whereas in other cases the ventricles are of normal size. Despite the absence of radiographic changes, these patients exhibit the clinical manifestations of shunt malfunction, as in the above case, and

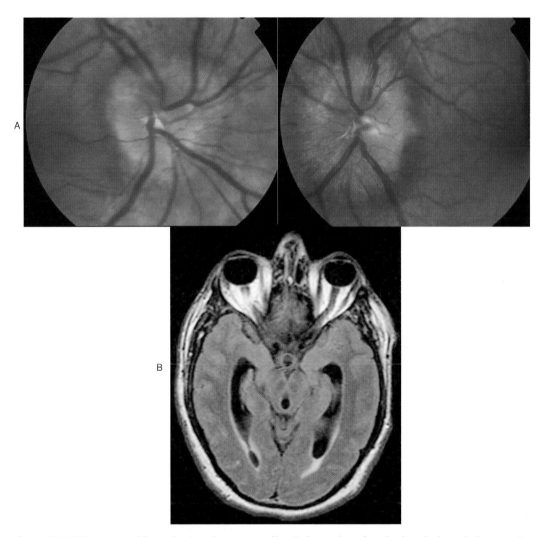

Figure 10.15 This 40-year-old man developed new onset of headaches and was found to have hydrocephalus secondary to decompensated aqueductal stenosis. (A) Fundus examination shows bilateral papilledema. (B) Axial FLAIR MR image shows moderate enlargement of the lateral and third ventricles with periventricular hyperintensity indicating subependymal CSF resorption. This characteristic radiographic sign of ventricular obstruction is not present in all cases.

should be treated accordingly. The challenge for the clinician in this setting is to hold firm to the conviction that the shunt is obstructed, based solely on the clinical findings.

Neuro-ophthalmic manifestations of hydrocephalus and shunt failure are varied. In addition to the dorsal midbrain syndrome, abnormal ocular motility may be due to sixth nerve paresis (unilateral or bilateral), third or fourth nerve paresis, skew deviation or see-saw nystagmus. Visual loss is most commonly due to papilledema (Figure 10.15A), but may also be caused by optic nerve or chiasmal compression or by occipital infarction due to occlusion of the posterior cerebral arteries (Figure 10.16,

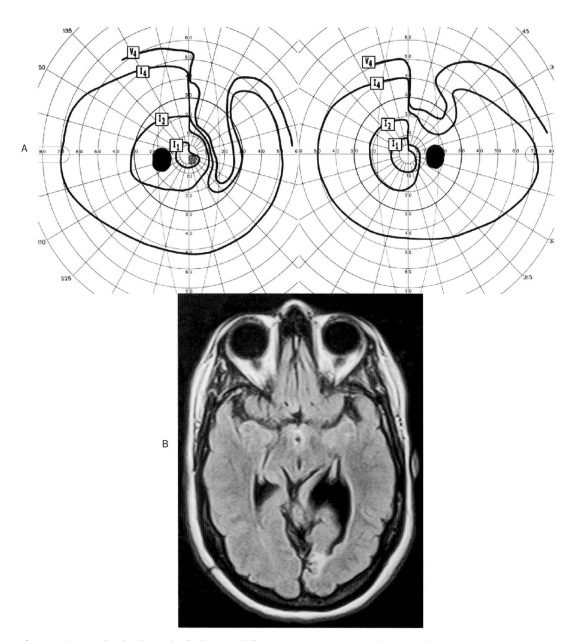

Figure 10.16 Visual and radiographic findings in a different patient with shunt malfunction. This young man with a ventriculoperitoneal shunt for Chiari II malformation presented with recurrent episodes of headache and syncope. The diagnosis of shunt malfunction was not appreciated for some time and in this interval he developed a small right homonymous visual field defect (A) due to proximal occipital infarction, seen here on axial FLAIR MR image (B).

see also Chapter 8, Constricted fields after herniation).

Diagnosis: Shunt malfunction in the absence of ventriculomegaly

Tip: The dorsal midbrain syndrome is an important and early sign of shunt failure and may occur even in the absence of radiographic changes.

FURTHER READING

Vitamin B12 deficiency

E. Andres, N. H. Loukili, E. Noel *et al.*, Vitamin B12 (cobalamin) deficiency in elderly patients. *Can Med Assoc J*, **171** (2004), 241–59.

R. Carmel, Current concepts in cobalamin deficiency. *Annu Rev Med*, **51** (2001), 357–8.

K. Juhasz-Pocsine, S. A. Rudnicki, R. L. Archer, S. I. Harik, Neurologic complications of gastric bypass surgery for morbid obesity. *Neurology*, **68** (2007), 1843–50.

J. Lindenbaum, E. B. Healton, D. C. Savage *et al.*, Neuropsychiatric disorders caused by cobalamin deficiency in the absence of anemia or macrocytosis. *N Engl J Med*, **318** (1988), 1720–8.

D. Milea, Blindness in a strict vegan. *N Engl J Med*, **342** (2000), 897–8.

J. F. Rizzo, Adenosine triphosphate deficiency: a genre of optic neuropathy. *Neurology*, **45** (1995), 11–16.

Digoxin toxicity

V. P. Butler Jr., J. G. Odel, E. Rath *et al.*, Digitalis-induced visual disturbances with therapeutic serum digitalis concentrations. *Ann Intern Med*, **123** (1995), 676–80.

H. A. Horst, K. D. Kolenda, G. Duncker, F. Schenck, H. Lottler, Color vision deficiencies induced by subtoxic and toxic digoxin and digitoxin serum levels. *Med Klin*, **83** (1988), 541–7.

J. R. Piltz, C. Wertenbaker, S. E. Lance, T. Slamovits, H. F. Leeper, Digoxin toxicity: recognizing the varied visual presentations. *J Clin Neuroophthalmol*, **13** (1993), 275–80.

R. G. Weleber, W. T. Shults, Digoxin retinal toxicity: clinical and electrophysiologic evaluation of a cone dysfunction syndrome. *Arch Ophthalmol*, **99** (1981), 1568–72.

Myasthenia

K. C. Golnik, R. Pena, A. G. Lee, E. R. Eggenberger, An ice test for the diagnosis of myasthenia gravis. *Ophthalmology*, **106** (1999), 1282–6.

E. B. Ing, S. Y. Ing, T. Ing, J. A. Ramocki, The complication rate of edrophonium testing for suspected myasthenia gravis. *Can J Ophthalmol*, **35** (2000), 141–4.

K. C. Kubis, H. V. Danesh-Meyer, P. J. Savino, R. C. Sergott, The ice test versus the rest test in myasthenia gravis. *Ophthalmology*, **107** (2000), 1995–8.

L. L. Kusner, A. Puwanat, H. J. Kaminski, Ocular myasthenia. Diagnosis, treatment and prognosis. *Neurologist*, **12** (2006), 231–9.

Aneurysmal third nerve palsy

S. Bracard, R. Anxionnat, L. Picard, Current diagnostic modalities for intracranial aneurysms. *Neuroimag Clin N Am*, **16** (2006), 397–411.

D. M. Jacobson, J. D. Trobe, The emerging role of magnetic resonance angiography in the management of patients with third cranial nerve palsy. *Am J Ophthalmol*, **128** (1999), 94–6.

M. J. Kupersmith, G. Heller, T. A. Cox, Magnetic resonance angiography and clinical evaluation of third nerve palsies and posterior communicating artery aneurysms. *J Neurosurg*, **105** (2006), 228–34.

A. G. Lee, L. A. Hayman, P. W. Brazis, The evaluation of isolated third nerve palsy revisited: an update on the evolving role of magnetic resonance, computed tomography and catheter angiography. *Surv Ophthalmol*, **47** (2002), 137–57.

R. M. MacFadzean, E. M. Teasdale, Computerized tomography angiography in isolated third nerve palsies. *J Neurosurg*, **88** (1998), 679–84.

One-and-a-half syndrome

M. R. Hanson, M. A. Hamid, R. L. Tomsak, S. S. Chou, R. J. Leigh, Selective saccadic palsy caused by pontine lesions: clinical, physiological and pathological correlations. *Ann Neurol*, **20** (1986), 209–17.

M. Wall, S. H. Wray, The one-and-a-half syndrome – a unilateral disorder of the pontine tegmentum: a study of 20 cases and review of the literature. *Neurology*, **33** (1983), 971–80.

Cortical visual loss with negative neuro-imaging

P. W. Brazis, A. G. Lee, N. Graff-Radford, N. P. Desai, E. R. Eggenberger, Homonymous visual field defects in patients without corresponding structural lesions on neuroimaging. *J Neuroophthalmol*, **20** (2000), 92–6.

D. G. Cogan, Visual disturbances with focal progressive dementing disease. *Am J Ophthalmol*, **100** (1985), 68–72.

R. T. Johnson, D. J. Gibbs, Creutzfeldt-Jakob disease and related transmissible spongiform encephalopathies. *N Eng J Med*, **339** (1998), 1994–2004.

K. Kallenberg, W. J. Schulz-Schaeffer, U. Jastrow *et al.*, Creutzfeldt-Jakob disease: comparative analysis of MR imaging sequences. *AJNR*, **27** (2006), 1459–62.

S. Kropp, W. J. Schulz-Schaeffer, M. Finkenstaedt *et al.*, The Heidenhain variant of Creutzfeldt-Jakob disease. *Arch Neurol*, **56** (1999), 55–61.

A. G. Lee, C. O. Martin, Neuro-ophthalmic findings in the visual variant of Alzheimer's disease. *Ophthalmology*, **111** (2004), 376–81.

E. Margolin, S. K. Gujar, J. D. Trobe, Isolated cortical visual loss with subtle brain MRI abnormalities in a case of hypoxic-ischemic encephalopathy. *J Neuroophthalmol*, **27** (2007), 292–6.

P. J. Nestor, D. Caine, T. D. Fryer, J. Clarke, J. R. Hodges, The topography of metabolic deficits in posterior cortical atrophy (the visual variant of Alzheimer's disease) with FDG-PET. *J Neurol Neurosurg Psychiatry* **74** (2003), 1521–9.

Skull base tumors with negative imaging

M. Ibrahim, H. Parmar, D. Gandhi, S. K. Mukherji, *J Neuro-ophthalmol*, **27** (2007), 129–37.

Shunt failure with negative neuro-imaging

J. J. Corbett, Neuro-ophthalmologic complications of hydrocephalus and shunting procedures. *Semin Neurol*, **6** (1986), 111–23.

D. M. Katz, J. D. Trobe, K. M. Muraszko, R. C. Dauser, Shunt failure without ventriculomegaly proclaimed by ophthalmic findings. *J Neurosurg*, **81** (1994), 721–5.

I. B. Mizrachi, J. D. Trobe, S. S. Gebarski, H. J. Garton, Papilledema in the assessment of ventriculomegaly. *J Neuroophthalmol*, **26** (2006), 260–3.

T.-N. Nguyen, R. C. Polomeno, J.-P. Farmer, J. L. Montes, Ophthalmic complications of slit-ventricle syndrome in children. *Ophthalmology*, **109** (2002), 520–5.

11

Over-ordering tests

Continued developments in ancillary testing, particularly in the field of neuro-imaging, have greatly enhanced the prompt and accurate diagnosis of a variety of neuro-ophthalmic disorders. As impressive as this technology is, there are still conditions in which information obtained from the history and physical examination is more valuable than the results of ancillary investigations. Unnecessary testing is to be discouraged for several reasons. Medical testing entails additional expense which can be considerable. Some forms of testing involve risk to the patient and certainly should be avoided if not truly necessary. Finally, the addition of extra testing can create a delay in diagnosis which may affect the outcome.

Testing should be limited to those conditions which could actually be responsible for the condition under investigation. While this may sound obvious, in clinical practice testing is often ordered as part of a "shotgun" approach to diagnosis that does not adhere to this principle. For example, a serum B12 level is sometimes obtained for patients with acute monocular visual loss. While B12 deficiency can indeed cause optic neuropathy, the clinical syndrome is that of symmetric, bilateral, subacute, central visual loss (see Chapter 10, Unexplained visual loss). Deficiency of vitamin B12 can cause a range of neurologic deficits but acute unilateral visual loss is not among them, and so this test should not be part of the work-up. In this chapter we highlight several examples of excessive ancillary testing.

Isolated unilateral mydriasis

Case: A 30-year-old paralegal developed blurred near vision and a mild ache behind the left eye. The next day she noticed that her left pupil was larger than the right pupil. She was otherwise healthy with no headache, diplopia, ptosis, other neurologic deficits or recent systemic symptoms. Physical examination in a local emergency room was unrevealing except for a large, unreactive left pupil. A head CT was normal as were a subsequent MRI and MRA. A cerebral arteriogram was recommended but the patient was sent first for neuro-ophthalmic consultation.

Examination one week after symptom onset showed uncorrected visual acuity of 20/20 at distance in each eye. Near vision tested with Jaeger acuity was decreased to J8 OS compared to J1 OD, but could be improved to J1 using a +2.00 lens. Eye movements were full with brisk and accurate saccades, she was orthophoric in all fields of gaze and there was no ptosis. The right pupil measured 6 mm in dim room light and constricted briskly to 3 mm with direct light stimulation. The left pupil was 7 mm in dim room light and showed no apparent reaction to direct or consensual light stimulation. Pupillary reactivity in the left eye was not better when the patient viewed a near target. High-magnification slit-lamp examination of the left eye showed paralysis of most of the iris sphincter except for two focal segments that were briskly reactive to light stimulation.

This patient's acute unilateral mydriasis raised the possibility of third nerve palsy due to a posterior communicating artery aneurysm, and the work-up was directed with this possibility in mind. Can isolated mydriasis, in fact, be a sign of a posterior communicating artery aneurysm?

There are no documented cases of a posterior communicating artery (pCOM) aneurysm that presented as isolated pupillary dilation. The fibers that subserve pupillomotor innervation travel on the dorsal medial surface of the oculomotor nerve and in this location are vulnerable to compression by an aneurysm at the junction of the posterior communicating and the internal carotid arteries. As a result of this anatomic relationship, pupillary dilation can be an early sign of aneurysmal compression. However, in such cases there is virtually always involvement of other third nerve motor fibers. The caveat in applying this "rule" is that one must perform an ocular motor examination that is adequate to rule out other elements of third nerve dysfunction. Specifically, it is not sufficient to simply ask the patient about diplopia or look only for ductional deficits on examination. Cross-cover testing should be performed, particularly on upgaze and with the suspect eye in adduction to rule out subtle underaction of the elevators and of the medial rectus muscle, respectively. In addition, external examination should include careful inspection of lid position and function. If other evidence of third nerve palsy has been excluded in this way, one can be confident that the unilateral mydriasis is an isolated finding and is not due to compression by a pCOM aneurysm.

If an isolated, enlarged and poorly reactive pupil is not a sign of a pCOM aneurysm, what other causes should be considered?

There are other causes of third nerve palsy that can produce isolated pupillary dilation, but they are rare. For example, a small mesencephalic hemorrhage affecting the fascicular pathway of the third nerve can cause isolated mydriasis. In transtentorial herniation, pupillary dilation may be the first sign of third nerve compromise, but in such cases alteration of consciousness is also present.

More commonly, the site of pathology is peripheral: injury to the short ciliary nerves in the orbit (an Adie's tonic pupil), pharmacologic blockade of the iris or direct damage to the iris sphincter muscle. Sphincter muscle damage may result from trauma, inflammation or ischemia. Evidence of previous trauma or inflammation can generally be seen with slit-lamp examination. Causes of iris ischemia include giant cell arteritis, high-grade carotid stenosis and angle closure glaucoma. An iris sphincter that is pharmacologically blocked by an atropinic substance is usually widely dilated and fails to constrict to full-strength (1% to 4%) pilocarpine.

This patient's slit-lamp examination showed no structural abnormalities of the iris, leaving tonic pupil and pharmacologic blockade as the primary considerations. Following instillation of dilute ($\frac{1}{8}$%) pilocarpine, the left pupil constricted from 7 mm to 4 mm, consistent with cholinergic denervation supersensitivity. The right pupil was unchanged. The patient received a diagnosis of Adie's tonic pupil and was managed expectantly. Examination three months later showed no improvement of the pupillary response to light in the left eye but there was now a slow, sustained constriction during near effort. One year later the left pupil was 1 mm smaller than the right in dim light but still showed minimal response to light stimulation.

Discussion: The pathophysiology of an Adie's tonic pupil is a two-fold process, acutely reflecting the effects of *denervation*, and later those of *reinnervation*. In the acute stage of denervation, the iris sphincter and ciliary muscle are paralyzed. The patient complains of photophobia and blurred near vision. The pupil is dilated and unresponsive to both light stimulation and near effort, and accommodation is lost. Denervation is typically incomplete, manifest as incomplete or sectoral palsy of the iris sphincter (see Chapter 9, Acute tonic pupil vs. pharmacologic mydriasis).

Supersensitivity of the iris sphincter to weak cholinergic agonists develops within several days to

Table 11.1 Features of an Adie's pupil

Day 1:	Large pupil size in darkness and in bright light
	Unresponsive to light stimulation and to near effort
	Sectoral palsy of the iris sphincter (seen under magnification)
Week 1:	Cholinergic denervation supersensitivity to dilute pilocarpine
Week 8:	Light-near dissociation
	Slow, sustained (tonic) pupillary constriction during and after near effort
Month 6:	Baseline pupil size in room light begins to decrease

weeks following denervation injury. The most commonly used pharmacologic agent for demonstrating such supersensitivity is dilute ($\frac{1}{8}$%) pilocarpine. This solution can be made by drawing up 0.1 cc of 1% pilocarpine with 0.7 cc of sterile saline in a 1 cc tuberculin syringe. The proposed criterion for a positive response is either (1) the affected pupil constricts 0.5 mm more than the unaffected pupil or (2) the suspected pupil, which was larger than the normal pupil before instillation of pilocarpine, becomes the smaller pupil after instillation. Denervation supersensitivity can be demonstrated in about 80% of patients with an Adie's pupil but takes several days to develop (Table 11.1). It is important to note that occasional patients with a dilated pupil from a third nerve palsy (i.e. preganglionic denervation) may also exhibit such supersensitivity. Therefore, the presence of cholinergic supersensitivity is not definitive evidence of an Adie's pupil but must be taken into consideration with the other clinical findings.

In the reinnervation stage, the short ciliary nerves regenerate and reconnect to their end organs. The relative abundance of resprouting accommodative fibers leads to recovery of accommodation (near vision). In addition, accommodative fibers mistakenly make connections to the iris sphincter. This aberrant reinnervation leads to recovery of pupillary constriction when focusing at near but

with a slow and delayed (tonic) movement. Because the number of surviving pupilloconstrictor fibers is sparse, the pupillary light reflex remains poor or absent. This combination of a poor pupil light reflex with good near response is termed *light-near dissociation*.

Tonic pupils may occur from a variety of local processes affecting the ciliary ganglion, such as orbital trauma (accidental or iatrogenic), tumor, ischemia or infection. Tonic pupils may also occur as a manifestation of a more widespread autonomic process, such as diabetic or alcoholic peripheral neuropathy, and in these cases both pupils are affected. However, most cases of tonic pupil occur as a spontaneous unilateral condition, usually in women between the ages of 20 and 50 years and it is this idiopathic form that has been termed an *Adie's tonic pupil*. When diminished muscle stretch reflexes are an associated finding, the condition is called Adie or Holmes–Adie syndrome. Neuro-imaging is not indicated for the patient with a typical Adie's pupil.

Diagnosis: Adie's tonic pupil

Tip: For practical purposes, isolated unilateral pupillary dilation in an alert and neurologically intact patient is *not* a sign of third nerve compression. Likely causes are Adie's tonic pupil or pharmacologic mydriasis.

Acute unilateral visual loss with disc edema

Case: A 62-year-old farmer awoke with decreased vision in the left eye. Specifically, he described darkening of the bottom half of vision in that eye unassociated with head or eye pain, photopsias, other focal neurologic deficits or systemic symptoms. His medical history was positive for hypertension and hyperlipidemia. Three weeks earlier an additional anti-hypertensive medication had been added. Five days after onset, examination showed visual acuity of 20/25 OD and 20/40 OS with a 2+ left RAPD. Goldmann perimetry demonstrated an inferior altitudinal defect in the left eye and a full field in the right eye (Figure 11.1A). Fundus examination

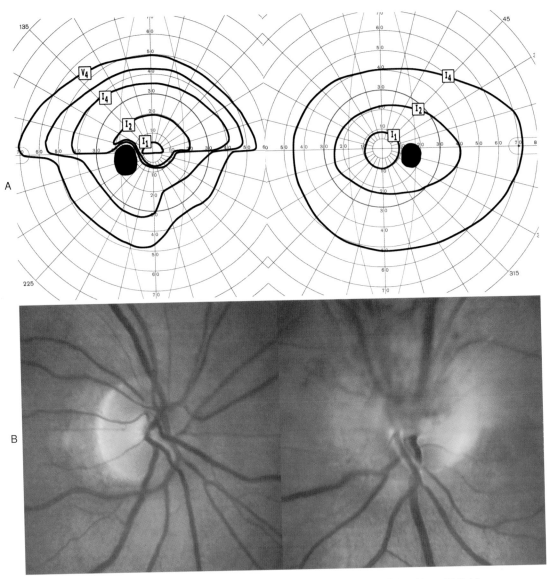

Figure 11.1 Examination findings in the above 62-year-old farmer with acute unilateral visual loss. (A) Goldmann perimetry shows an inferior altitudinal defect in the left eye; the field in the right eye is full. (B) Fundus photographs taken five days after onset of visual loss show segmental disc edema superiorly in the left eye; the right disc appears normal and has a small cup.

showed swelling of the superior half of the left optic disc; the right disc was normal in appearance but "crowded", with a small physiologic cup (Figure 11.1B).

Additional testing included an MRI of brain and orbits with contrast, a cranial MRA, carotid Dopplers, a transthoracic echocardiogram, visual evoked potential, and a variety of blood tests for coagulopathy, all of which were normal or negative. One month later, disc edema had resolved leaving superior pallor, but his visual field defect was unchanged.

Can you diagnose the cause of this patient's acute monocular visual loss based on the clinical findings? Are ancillary tests needed?

This patient presented with an acute, painless, unilateral optic neuropathy with altitudinal field loss and corresponding segmental disc edema. These clinical findings are sufficiently characteristic of non-arteritic anterior ischemic optic neuropathy (NAION) that little ancillary testing is needed. Specifically, cranial, carotid and cardiac imaging are not likely to add anything relevant to management decisions.

Discussion: NAION is a relatively common disorder, typically affecting middle-aged and older individuals. Visual loss is usually painless and often present upon awakening. An inferior altitudinal defect is the most common pattern of visual loss, frequently with preservation of normal visual acuity. Optic disc edema may be diffuse or segmental and peri-papillary splinter hemorrhages are common. Visual loss is most often maximal at onset, but up to one-third of patients experience further decline of vision over the next 10 days, termed progressive NAION. Once disc edema has resolved, usually within a few weeks, further visual loss is highly unlikely. Some modest improvement of visual acuity is common in the months following an episode of NAION but visual field defects are typically permanent. A repeat episode in the same eye is rare; however, 15 to 25% of patients will experience a similar attack in the fellow eye in the future.

The pathogenesis of NAION is multifactorial, including some degree of atherosclerosis and an underlying predisposing optic disc structure. Patients with NAION typically have a crowded optic disc with little or no physiologic cup, termed a "disc-at-risk". In addition to these predisposing factors, recent interest has focused on the role of systemic

hypotension in the pathogenesis of this disorder. Occasionally episodes of profound hypotension (e.g. cardiac arrest) precipitate ischemic optic neuropathy. In addition, a possible role of less cataclysmic nocturnal hypotension, particularly that induced by anti-hypertensive medication taken in the evening, has been posited in the pathogenesis of this disorder. Other mechanisms that may contribute to optic nerve infarction in certain cases include vasospasm, loss of local autoregulation, and the metabolic and circulatory changes that occur in sleep apnea syndrome. Acquired and hereditary coagulopathies are not usually identified in patients with NAION, though such factors may play a role in occasional patients under age 50 years who lack the usual predisposing conditions.

Notably absent from the above list of etiologic factors are carotid artery disease and emboli. In contrast to vaso-occlusive events in the retinal circulation, NAION is rarely the result of embolic occlusion. Due to the branching pattern of the ocular circulation, emboli entering the ophthalmic artery are likely to proceed via laminar flow to the central or branch retinal arteries. In contrast, the posterior ciliary arteries emerge more at right angles from the ophthalmic artery and are therefore not susceptible to emboli. While rare cases of ischemic optic neuropathy secondary to complete carotid occlusion, carotid dissection or emboli have been reported, it is important to note that carotid artery disease has *not* been found in a higher percentage of patients with NAION as compared to age-matched controls. When carotid artery stenosis is found in a patient with NAION, it is just as likely to involve the contralateral side as the side with the visual loss. Specific features that suggest carotid artery disease may have played a role in an episode of NAION include preceding transient monocular visual loss, dimming of vision with changes of posture or exertion, ipsilateral pain and associated Horner syndrome, and in these settings carotid ultrasonography may be appropriate. In the large majority of patients with NAION, however, carotid artery imaging is not indicated. If carotid imaging is obtained in a patient with NAION and hemodynamically significant blockage is found, it should be considered in the category of asymptomatic carotid stenosis.

The diagnosis of NAION is a clinical one; in most cases few ancillary tests are needed. In addition to the investigation of risk factors for vascular disease, the main focus of laboratory testing in such patients is the identification of those patients with the arteritic variety of AION (see Chapter 12, Evaluation and treatment of giant cell arteritis).

Diagnosis: Non-arteritic anterior ischemic optic neuropathy (NAION)

Tip: NAION is due to small vessel disease involving the optic disc. In typical cases, investigation for an embolic source is not indicated.

Acute isolated sixth nerve palsy

Case: A 69-year-old retired fireman with stable hypertension and hyperlipidemia noticed double vision and minor aching behind his left eye while at a family reunion. He mentioned his symptoms to his wife who noticed nothing unusual about his appearance. Over the next two days his left eye turned noticeably inward but he still had no other neurologic or systemic symptoms. Examination now showed a moderate esotropia and loss of abduction in the left eye (Figure 11.2). Left lateral rectus saccades were markedly slow. Optic nerve function and appearance were normal, as were pupils, lids and other cranial nerves, and there was no evidence of orbitopathy.

What is the most likely diagnosis and what evaluation would be appropriate?

An acute microvascular sixth nerve palsy was diagnosed. The natural course and excellent prognosis associated with a vasculopathic ocular motor neuropathy were explained to the patient and his wife. The option of ordering an MR scan was also discussed but not recommended by the treating physician. Instead the patient was advised to return for re-evaluation one week later. A CBC, ESR and C-reactive protein were obtained, results of which were normal. At follow-up one week later his periorbital ache was resolved, but the abduction deficit was unchanged. Other neurologic findings were again normal. Over the next eight weeks, the patient demonstrated spontaneous and complete recovery of his sixth nerve palsy.

Discussion: Etiologies of acute sixth nerve palsy include tumor, stroke, demyelinating disease, intracranial hemorrhage, meningeal disease, increased intracranial pressure, trauma and a variety of infectious, inflammatory and immunologic disorders. In many of these conditions there are other neurologic deficits and/or systemic symptoms. An acute, *isolated* sixth nerve palsy in adults older than age 50 years is most commonly due to microvascular ischemia of the peripheral portion of the nerve, commonly referred to as an *ischemic* or *vasculopathic* cranial neuropathy. Such palsies are usually accompanied by ipsilateral headache or retrobulbar pain that may precede the palsy by a day or two and usually remits in 7 to 10 days. The motor deficit in vasculopathic cranial neuropathies (third, fourth and sixth) often shows initial progression for

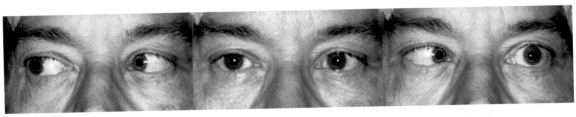

Figure 11.2 Motility examination in a 69-year-old retired fireman with an acute left sixth nerve palsy. The eyes are esotropic in primary position and there is no abduction of the left eye past midline.

several days, occurring in about 50% of patients. It is helpful to recognize that this is a common feature of the natural history of this disorder and, as long as other features are typical, does not warrant additional investigation. While ancillary testing can be obtained to exclude other etiologies, the diagnosis of a vasculopathic sixth nerve palsy is a clinical one, based on the following criteria: age greater than 50 years, one or more vascular risk factors, absence of neurologic signs and symptoms other than initial ipsilateral headache, and spontaneous recovery which is usually complete within four months. In cases with typical clinical findings, little additional testing is needed. Assessment of vascular risk factors (blood pressure, serum glucose and lipid profile) should be undertaken. In patients older than 60 years of age, serologic tests for giant cell arteritis should be obtained. In patients without associated pain, a Tensilon (edrophonium chloride) test may be performed. Some clinicians obtain an MRI in such patients; others opt for observational management, as in the above case. More extensive testing, however (e.g. lumbar puncture, carotid imaging, evoked potentials and additional blood tests), is unnecessary and should be discouraged.

Serial examinations are critically important in the evaluation of an acute and isolated sixth nerve palsy. The specific goals in such evaluation are assuring that the palsy remains isolated, and documenting the expected spontaneous recovery. The determination of improvement should be based on examination findings, as patients are notoriously unreliable at assessing improvement of their motility deficit. The degree of sixth nerve dysfunction can be objectively assessed as degrees of abduction past midline, millimeters of scleral show on abduction compared to the fellow eye, or prism diopters of esotropia in primary position. Spontaneous recovery is the clinical feature that best defines this syndrome. Continued progression beyond two weeks, failure to show some improvement by eight weeks or significant residual nerve palsy after six months should cast doubt upon the diagnosis and prompt additional evaluation. In addition, any patient with

a history of cancer should undergo prompt evaluation, particularly neuro-imaging.

This restrained approach to the evaluation of a sixth nerve palsy applies to an *acute* event. In contrast, any patient with a chronic ocular motor palsy (usually defined as duration greater than six months) should be thoroughly evaluated for a compressive lesion at the skull base, meningeal infiltration and increased intracranial pressure (Figure 11.3). It should be noted that this principle is different from the approach used in many other medical situations in which chronicity confers a sense of the benign nature of the disease process.

The diagnosis of a vasculopathic third nerve palsy is somewhat more complex, relying on the pattern of motor and parasympathetic nerve involvement in addition to other clinical features as described above. Because the fibers that subserve pupillary constriction are located peripherally on the nerve, the pupil in vasculopathic third nerve palsy is often spared, due to vascular supply to this area by pial arterial branches. In contrast, in third nerve palsy due to a pCOM aneurysm, pupillary dysfunction is an early and frequent finding. The state of the pupil is therefore helpful in distinguishing vasculopathic from aneurysmal mechanisms, and has been summarized in the statement "a third nerve palsy with pupil sparing is not due to a pCOM aneurysm". An important exception to this "rule of the pupil", however, is the patient in whom the third nerve palsy is partial, i.e. in addition to pupil sparing, one or more extraocular muscles are spared as well. Such partial pupil-sparing third nerve palsy is indeed occasionally produced by aneurysmal compression. Thus, in cases of partial palsy, the presence of pupil-sparing is less reassuring, and some form of neuro-imaging is appropriate to rule out an aneurysm (see Chapter 10, Headache and third nerve palsy). In the adult patient with an otherwise complete but pupil-sparing third nerve palsy with vascular risk factors, ancillary testing is usually considered optional.

There is no specific treatment for a vasculopathic cranial nerve palsy. Symptomatic relief of diplopia can be achieved by patching, occlusive tape on one lens or application of a paste-on prism. Insofar as

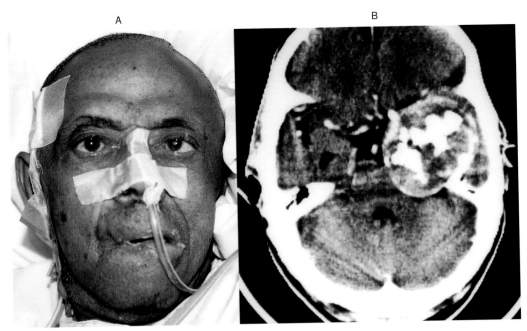

Figure 11.3 (A) Patient who suffered an acute left middle cerebral artery stroke. He had been followed for a chronic left sixth nerve palsy for the preceding 10 years but without neuro-imaging. In addition to his esotropia, notice his left Horner syndrome and right central facial weakness. (B) Axial post-contrast CT shows a giant, partially thrombosed, left intracavernous internal carotid artery aneurysm.

a vasculopathic palsy is a marker for atherosclerotic disease, daily aspirin is appropriate as prophylaxis for other ischemic events such as stroke and heart attack. Some patients experience a subsequent similar episode involving the same cranial nerve, another ocular motor nerve or a facial palsy. Even in the case of such recurrence, the prognosis for ultimate recovery is excellent.

Diagnosis: Vasculopathic cranial mononeuropathy

Tip: The diagnosis of a vasculopathic cranial nerve palsy is a clinical one. Ancillary testing should be reserved for patients with an atypical clinical course.

Episodic scintillating scotoma

Case: A 55-year-old teacher had experienced several episodes of transient binocular visual loss over the past two years. She described "shimmering" vision that began close to fixation and spread out to the periphery over 20 minutes. Most of these episodes occurred in the right hemifield, but occasional attacks were on the left. There were no other focal deficits, altered consciousness or headache associated with the visual loss. She was generally in good health and taking no medications. She reported a remote history of "sick headaches" without visual disturbance that were usually associated with menses and remitted in her late twenties after her first pregnancy. Her neurologic examination was normal including visual fields full to confrontational testing.

Does this patient need neuro-imaging? An EEG? Other investigation?

The slow spread of the scintillations across the visual field described by this patient is considered pathognomonic of migraine. The fact that her visual disturbance sometimes switches sides further rules out a structural lesion. In this case, no additional testing is needed.

Discussion: Migraine with or without visual aura is extremely common, with a lifetime prevalence of 12 to 33% in women and 4 to 22% in men. Many patients with migraine present to primary care physicians, others to ophthalmologists, neurologists or other healthcare providers. Not all patients with migraine require neuro-imaging or other ancillary testing and it is helpful for the clinician to have a set of guidelines for deciding when such work-up is needed.

The presence or absence of headache is not a useful criterion since migraine visual aura without headache is a common occurrence, termed *acephalgic migraine* or *migraine equivalent* in the older literature. Moreover, 20% of vertebrobasilar transient ischemic attacks and even occasional seizures are accompanied by headache. The temporal and spatial characteristics of the visual episode are much more helpful. As noted previously (see Chapter 1, Twinkling scotoma), migrainous visual phenomena are usually positive (i.e. seeing something that is *not* there rather than not seeing something that *is* there) and usually include a quality of motion (shimmering, sparkling or vibrating). These migrainous scintillations often start adjacent to fixation and spread to the periphery on one side over 20 minutes (Figure 11.4). This slow spread or "march" corresponds to the speed of the spreading cortical depression that underlies an attack and is generally considered to be pathognomonic for migraine. There are rare cases in which this characteristic pattern of scintillations has been associated with a structural lesion (specifically, an occipital arteriovenous malformation or tumor), and it is believed that in these individuals a mechanical stimulus has provoked an episode of migraine. A helpful tip-off in such rare cases is the fact that attacks occur exclusively in the same hemifield. About 20% of patients with migraine report their attacks as always being on the same side (termed

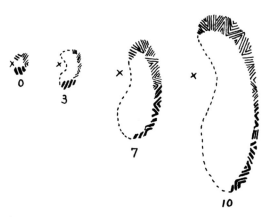

Figure 11.4 Migraine visual aura. Typical scintillating scotoma is shown at varying time intervals after onset. The "X" in each instance indicates the visual fixation point and the numbers represent minutes. (From K. S. Lashley, *Arch Neurol Psychiatr,* **46** (1941), 331–9, with permission.)

"side-locked" migraine), so this feature alone does not guarantee the presence of a structural lesion but the converse is very helpful: attacks that switch sides are *not* due to an underlying mass lesion.

Migraine attacks are frequently precipitated by an internal or external trigger, and eliciting this history can be helpful in diagnosis as well as treatment. Stress and hormonal change are the most common triggers. The actual migraine episode typically occurs not during the period of stress but in the letdown phase that follows. Hormonal triggers most often involve a decline in estrogen levels such as just prior to menses and during peri-menopause when estrogen secretion tends to be erratic. Other triggers include skipping meals, sleeping late, strong smells, bright lights, caffeine withdrawal and certain foods. In some cases, more than one trigger is required to precipitate an episode; for example, missing breakfast and coffee because one is running late for a morning appointment. In its full-fledged form the headache is severe and associated with nausea, vomiting and a heightened sensitivity to light and sound; however not all migraine attacks have these characteristics. Migraine headaches are usually relieved by sleep and often by triptan medications. In the vast majority of cases, the focal deficit of a migraine attack (usually visual, occasionally sensory or motor) resolves completely within 30 to 60 minutes. More prolonged persistence of a focal deficit suggests an ischemic complication or the possibility of a different underlying cause. If a patient thinks that vision has not fully returned to normal after an episode, and in cases with other atypical features, it is important to obtain visual field testing to look for a persistent defect.

The definition of migraine includes the tendency to have recurrent attacks; it is not possible to make a diagnosis of migraine based on a single episode. The clinician should be extremely careful when attributing a patient's symptoms to a first migraine attack, especially considering that the typical symptoms, namely headache, nausea and vomiting, are the same as those of increased intracranial pressure, meningitis and subarachnoid hemorrhage. For a patient with a first episode of isolated visual loss not accompanied by headache, neuro-imaging is not indicated if the clinical features of the attack are typical.

Putting together these clinical features, the indications for neurodiagnostic investigation in a patient with suspected migraine should include: a prolonged visual field defect or other persistent focal neurologic deficit and attacks always localized to the same area. A recent change in pattern (frequency, duration or quality) without explanation (i.e. a change in trigger factors) should also prompt additional testing. The above patient illustrates a common change in pattern: women who have migraine headaches in their teens and twenties often find that their headaches resolve with pregnancy but migraine recurs during peri-menopause in the form of visual aura without headache. In patients with recurrent episodes and typical clinical features, ancillary testing is not needed.

Diagnosis: Migraine aura

Tip: The slow spread of photopsias across the visual field is the most distinctive feature indicating migraine as the cause of transient binocular visual loss.

Unexplained visual loss

Case: A 19-year-old college student experienced new onset of headaches and episodes of transient visual loss during midterm exams. Following one of her episodes the vision in her left eye failed to return. She described total blackness of vision and on examination claimed she was barely able to see light in that eye. Fundus appearance was normal bilaterally, as were all tests of vision in her right eye including normal visual field by confrontation. Pupillary responses were brisk and symmetric with no RAPD. An MRI of brain and orbits and a variety of blood tests were unrevealing. Her headaches persisted and two weeks later vision in her left eye remained bare light perception.

What feature in this case suggests non-organic visual loss? Is additional ancillary testing needed?

This degree of visual loss (near-complete blindness in one eye) with clear ocular media is incompatible with a normal pupillary response and strongly suggests non-organic visual loss. Visual acuity was re-measured using crossed cylinders to fog the vision in the patient's right eye. With the fellow eye so blurred that she could only be reading with the "bad" left eye, she was able to easily and accurately read the entire eye chart from the large E down to the 20/20 line. Based on this observation, a diagnosis of non-organic visual loss was made. She was reassured that her vision would return to normal and received treatment for her tension-vascular headaches.

Discussion: Non-organic (functional) visual loss is a common neuro-ophthalmic problem, encompassing malingering (feigned loss) and hysteria (also referred to as a conversion disorder). This diagnosis should be suspected when the clinical findings are inconsistent with each other or when symptoms or signs do not conform to recognized disease patterns. Visual loss may affect one or both eyes, and ranges from mild to profound. The non-organic nature of the visual loss is most easily demonstrated when one eye is severely affected, typically by using techniques that "fog" the fellow eye, as in the case under discussion. In the crossed cylinder method, minus and plus cylinders of equal magnitudes are aligned in a trial frame over the "good" eye so that they cancel out optically. The patient is asked to read the Snellen chart with both eyes open, starting from the largest letters and reading down to the smallest. As the patient proceeds, the examiner turns one of the cylinders until the good eye is sufficiently blurred that the patient could only be reading with the eye that has the unexplained visual loss. Similar fogging can be achieved with increasing plus lenses in the phoropter, but with that technique the examiner loses the opportunity to observe the patient during the test and, in addition, the movement of the lenses is less subtle than the motion of the crossed cylinders. Red-green duochrome lenses can provide similar information, but in most cases the best acuity one can obtain with this method is around 20/40. Measurement of stereo-acuity can be a helpful adjunct for determining intact near vision. In cases involving both eyes or in those with visual loss in an only good eye, fogging techniques are not applicable. In such cases it is often possible to demonstrate better vision by working from the smallest letters on the Snellen chart up, using encouragement and the power of suggestion.

In cases of non-organic visual loss, the ideal test is one that demonstrates normal vision, but sometimes we must settle instead for showing gross inconsistencies. Examples of this include the ability to navigate about the room or reach for objects despite claimed blindness, intact central visual field in the face of severe loss of acuity, and apparent total monocular blindness with an intact pupillary response.

Diagnosis: Non-organic visual loss

Tip: In most cases of non-organic visual loss, specific examination techniques can disclose the nature of the disorder and thereby obviate the need for extensive and costly evaluation.

FURTHER READING

Adie's tonic pupil

D. M. Jacobson, Pupillary responses to dilute pilocarpine in preganglionic 3rd nerve disorders. *Neurology*, **40** (1990), 804–8.

R. H. Kardon, J. J. Corbett, H. S. Thompson, Segmental denervation and reinnervation of the iris sphincter as shown by infrared videographic transillumination. *Ophthamology*, **105** (1998), 313–21.

A. Kawasaki, Disorders of pupillary function, accommodation and lacrimation. In N. R. Miller, N. J. Newman, V. Biousse, J. B. Kerrison, eds., *Walsh and Hoyt's Clinical Neuro-Ophthalmology*, 6th edn. Philadelphia: Lippincott Williams and Wilkins, 2005, Vol. 1, Chapter 16, pp. 739–805.

Non-arteritic anterior ischemic optic neuropathy

A. C. Arnold, Pathogenesis of nonarteritic anterior ischemic optic neuropathy. *Ophthalmol Clin N Am*, **14** (2001), 83–98.

S. Lessell, Nonarteritic anterior ischemic optic neuropathy: enigma variations. *Arch Ophthalmol*, **117** (1999), 386–8.

V. Purvin, Ischemic optic neuropathy. *Semin Cerebrovasc Dis Stroke*, **4** (2004), 2–17.

Vasculopathic cranial mononeuropathy

K. L. Chou, S. L. Galetta, G. T. Liu *et al.*, Acute ocular motor mononeuropathies: prospective study of the roles of neuroimaging and clinical assessment. *J Neurol Sci*, **219** (2004), 35–9.

D. M. Jacobson, Progressive ophthalmoplegia with acute ischemic abducens nerve palsies. *Am J Ophthalmol*, **122** (1996), 278–9.

D. M. Jacobson, T. D. McCanna, P. M. Layde, Risk factors for ischemic ocular motor palsies. *Arch Ophthalmol*, **112** (1994), 961–6.

J. T. Kissel, R. M. Burde, T. G. Klingele, H. E. Zeiger, Pupil-sparing oculomotor palsies with internal carotid-posterior communicating artery aneurysms. *Ann Neurol*, **13** (1983), 149–54.

S. K. Sanders, A. Kawasaki, V. Purvin, Long-term prognosis in patients with vasculopathic sixth nerve palsy. *Am
J Ophthalmol*, **134** (2002), 81–4.

J. D. Trobe, Third nerve palsy and the pupil: footnotes to the
rule. *Arch Ophthalmol*, **106** (1988), 601–2.

Migraine

R. A. Davidoff. *Migraine. Manifestations, Pathogenesis, and
Management*, 2nd edn. Oxford: Oxford University Press,
2002.

S. L. Hupp, L. B. Kline, J. J. Corbett, Visual disturbances of
migraine. *Surv Ophthalmol*, **33** (1989), 221–36.

Non-organic visual loss

K. K. Kramer, F. G. La Piana, B. Appleton, Ocular malingering and hysteria: diagnosis and management. *Surv Ophthalmol*, **24** (1979), 89–96.

B. W. Miller, A review of practical tests for ocular malingering and hysteria. *Surv Ophthamol*, **17** (1973), 241–6.

H. S. Thompson, Functional visual loss. *Am J Ophthalmol*,
100 (1985), 209–13.

12

Management misadventures

Neuro-ophthalmologists are sometimes accused of concentrating on elucidation of the disease process with little emphasis on treatment, referred to by one of our colleagues as "admiring the disease rather than curing it". While we share our patients' frustration over the conditions that we cannot cure, we would dispute this view of what we do, sometimes termed "therapeutic nihilism". There are conditions in which intervention clearly makes a difference and we would be remiss if we did not highlight some of these situations.

Medical decisions frequently must be made on the basis of incomplete or ambiguous information, a fact of clinical practice that surely adds to our stress as clinicians. Ideally, we would have statistically significant results of multi-center trials and case-based analyses of the literature, but this kind of data is often lacking. Furthermore, practice parameters and recommendations regarding treatment evolve over time, as our understanding of disease process expands and additional information becomes available. Thus, what appears to be the correct course of action at one time may later be seen as ineffective or actually contraindicated. For example, neuromyelitis optica (Devic's disease) was, at one time, considered a subtype of multiple sclerosis, and patients were treated accordingly. More recently, this condition has emerged as a separate autoimmune entity in which the pathology, diagnostic markers and natural history are disparate from multiple sclerosis. Based on this additional information, it is no longer considered standard practice to treat patients with neuromyelitis optica using multiple sclerosis protocols.

We recognize that treatment recommendations are therefore not absolute, and are cautious about criticizing management decisions made by others. However, in some situations there are either enough data or sufficient collective clinical experience to recommend a particular course of action over another. In this chapter we look at a few such clinical scenarios. We have tried to emphasize those aspects of management in which there is some consensus and to downplay those that remain controversial.

Management of idiopathic intracranial hypertension

Case: A 26-year-old cashier presented with a one-month history of daily headaches and pulsatile tinnitus. For the past two weeks she had also experienced brief episodes in which her vision would gray out in both eyes, often precipitated by postural change. She was generally healthy but had been obese since high school and reported an additional 25 pound weight gain since she stopped smoking six months earlier.

Visual acuity was 20/20 in each eye with normal color vision, pupillary responses and ocular motility, and fundus examination showed severe bilateral optic disc edema. Her general neurologic examination was otherwise normal as was an MRI with contrast. A lumbar puncture in the lateral decubitus position demonstrated an opening pressure of 380 mm of water with normal protein, glucose and cell count. A diagnosis of idiopathic intracranial hypertension (pseudotumor cerebri syndrome) was made and she was treated with oral acetazolamide 250 mg twice per day.

The patient returned for follow-up two weeks later reporting no improvement of symptoms. A lumbar puncture was again performed, this time showing an opening pressure of 300 mm of water. Her headaches improved for a few days but then resumed, along with more frequent and prolonged transient visual obscurations. She worried that she was allergic to the acetazolamide because it caused intense paresthesias, so she stopped the medication. At return visit two weeks later she described dimming of vision, more in the right eye than the left, in addition to episodic visual loss. A third lumbar puncture showed an opening pressure of 340 mm of water and she was then sent for neuro-ophthalmic consultation.

Goldmann perimetry showed bilateral inferonasal depression and generalized constriction, worse in the right eye. Acetazolamide was restarted at a higher dose (500 mg sustained release form twice daily), and furosemide (40 mg daily) and a potassium supplement were added. She was reassured that paresthesia was a normal side-effect of the medication that typically improves over time. One week later there was some improvement of the visual field in the left eye but mild worsening in the right eye. Acetazolamide was increased to 500 mg three times daily but the visual field in the right eye continued to worsen over the next month, prompting an optic nerve sheath fenestration in the right eye. Two weeks post-operatively, optic nerve function in the right eye was improved and the degree of papilledema was decreased in both eyes. It was not clear whether the improvement of disc edema in the unoperated eye was a consequence of the surgery or due to beneficial effects of the medications, but with stabilization of optic nerve function and only mild disc edema, no additional surgery was recommended. She was continued on acetazolamide and furosemide, the importance of weight reduction for the long-term management of this condition was discussed and the patient was referred to a nutritionist.

Discussion: In managing patients with IIH, the two primary goals of treatment should always be kept in mind: prevention of visual loss and relief of symptoms (usually headache). While reduction of intracranial pressure is one method of achieving these goals, it is not necessarily the primary aim of treatment. The focus should be on the *effects* of increased intracranial pressure (ICP), not the high pressure itself. This case illustrates several issues that commonly arise in the management of IIH.

In the large majority of cases, increased ICP is caused by weight gain and in such patients the ultimate effective treatment is weight reduction. Unfortunately, weight loss does not happen overnight; it is difficult to achieve and to sustain. Other therapeutic modalities for IIH can be divided into medical and surgical treatments. Medical treatments include acetazolamide and furosemide for lowering pressure, and amitryptyline, topiramate and various analgesics for symptomatic relief of headache. (Because of its pharmacologic similarity to acetazolamide, topiramate may also exert a beneficial effect on ICP but this has not yet been demonstrated.) Surgical options consist of optic nerve fenestration, cerebrospinal fluid diversion (lumboperitoneal or ventriculoperitoneal shunting) and bariatric procedures.

Although there are no randomized, controlled trials assessing the effectiveness of acetazolamide for IIH, experts in this area generally agree that this medication is effective and recommend it as a first line medical agent. However the recommended daily dosage varies. An early study that measured ICP during acetazolamide infusion found that a dose of 4 grams was required to significantly lower pressure, but few patients are able to tolerate this high a dose. From case series and clinical experience, lower doses of acetazolamide (1–2 grams daily) are associated with improvement of signs and symptoms in most patients. Use of the 500 mg sustained release formulation rather than the 250 mg tablets achieves higher drug levels and is actually better tolerated in most patients, presumably because it avoids the peaks and troughs of the short acting form. Paresthesia, especially around the mouth and hands, is a common side-effect. Patients should be warned about this side-effect before starting treatment as they are more likely to tolerate this discomfort if they understand that it is not an allergy or a sign that the dose is too high. It should be explained that paresthesia is distinct from a rash, which indicates drug allergy and is an indication to discontinue the medication. A prior history of sulfa allergy does not necessarily predict an adverse reaction to acetazolamide and is not a contraindication to treatment. The use of acetazolamide during the first trimester of pregnancy is discouraged but inadvertent use has not been associated with an increased risk of fetal malformation. If treatment with acetazolamide is not adequate, furosemide can be added, usually with the addition of a potassium supplement.

The majority of patients with IIH can be managed adequately with medication and weight loss, but a subset requires more aggressive treatment in the form of surgery. The usual indication for surgical intervention is progressive visual loss despite maximal medical management, as exemplified in the above case (Table 12.1). In occasional patients, visual loss is so severe at onset that a trial of medical management is not wise, and this too represents an indication for surgery. Intractable headache despite maximal medical management sometimes prompts surgical intervention, but there are usually other treatment options that are preferable for these patients. Specific concerns in this setting include the high incidence of persistent headaches even after technically successful shunting, and the relatively frequent need for shunt revision in these patients.

The specific indication for surgery helps to determine which procedure is chosen. When the indication is progressive visual loss, optic nerve sheath fenestration (ONSF) is often preferred. When persistent headache is the indication, shunting may be preferable since only about half of patients who undergo ONSF experience sustained improvement of headache. This remains an area of controversy and not all experts in the field agree with this recommendation. When shunting is undertaken, the ventriculoperitoneal (VP) route is emerging as a better choice than the lumboperitoneal (LP). Although the initial risk of placing a VP shunt is slightly higher, the lower revision rate and better access for using an externally programmable pressure device favor this route over LP shunting. VP shunting for IIH became a more viable option with the development of stereotactic CT guidance for shunt placement, and so there is less information on the long-term safety and efficacy of these shunts compared to the LP route. In a patient who presents with severe, acute visual loss the preferred surgical procedure is whichever one can be obtained most expediently. If a patient suffers subsequent visual loss following either procedure, the other one should be employed as well.

The third surgical option for the management of IIH is gastroplasty. Obviously, this is not an adequate strategy for patients with acute or impending visual loss, but it does appear to be effective for long-term management. In most cases, dramatic weight loss over the first six months following surgery brings significant improvement of signs and symptoms related to increased ICP.

Serial lumbar punctures have a limited role in the management of IIH. The relatively short duration of pressure-lowering limits its utility as a treatment modality. After the initial tap, serial lumbar punctures are rarely needed from a diagnostic standpoint since management is guided by the signs and symptoms of increased ICP rather than the degree of pressure elevation. Recall that the goal of treatment is

Table 12.1 Indications for surgical intervention in IIH

Progressive visual loss despite maximal medical therapy
Severe visual loss at presentation
Unreliable patients (poor follow-up or non-organic
  visual fields)
Patients who are unable to tolerate medication
Patients at high risk for hypotensive events (e.g. dialysis)

not a particular CSF pressure but rather managing the effects of pressure. If a patient is asymptomatic and has minimal or no papilledema then treatment is adequate, regardless of an actual opening pressure measurement. Repeated lumbar punctures sometimes have a role as a temporizing measure, for example in a pregnant patient with IIH (in whom treatment options are more limited) or while waiting to organize a more definitive approach (delay in availability of a surgeon).

Treatment decisions in IIH are guided largely by the severity of symptoms and the status of the optic nerve. At each visit, the frequency and severity of symptoms (headaches, pulsatile tinnitus, transient visual obscurations and diplopia) should be recorded. Fundus photographs are useful for documenting changes in disc appearance. Because loss of central vision is typically a *late* finding in IIH, regular assessment of the visual field is crucial. This is particularly important when optic disc swelling appears to be improving. Resolution of papilledema is generally taken to be a good sign, indicating improvement of axonal transport. However, progressive attrition of nerve fibers will also produce a similar lessening of disc edema. The only way to ensure that resolution of papilledema indicates recovery rather than progressive neuronal death is to quantify optic nerve function, including measurement of visual fields (Table 12.2).

Table 12.2 Common errors in the management of IIH

Delay in initiating treatment
Using serial lumbar punctures for routine management
Failure to monitor visual fields
Using inadequate doses of acetazolamide
Neglecting to warn patients about acetazolamide
   side-effects
Trusting spurious opening pressure measurement on
   fluoroscopy
Delay in moving from medical to surgical management
Failure to provide adequate counseling regarding weight
   reduction

Tip: Serial lumbar punctures have a limited role in the treatment of IIH. Optimal management should include regular assessment of visual field status and mindfulness regarding the goals of treatment, namely improvement of symptoms and protection of optic nerve function.

Evaluation and treatment of giant cell arteritis

Case: An 83-year-old, active widow who lived alone suddenly lost vision in her left eye. Examination that day revealed bare light perception vision in the left eye with marked swelling of the left optic disc (Figure 12.1). All findings in her right eye were normal. Review of systems revealed that she had not been well recently. Over a two-month period, she had developed generalized joint pain and stiffness that caused difficulty arising from bed and participating in her daily fitness class. She had also noted scalp tingling and facial tenderness that was so severe that she could not comfortably rest her head on a pillow. Her jaw ached after taking more than two bites of food and everything had a metallic taste. She had lost several pounds due to poor appetite and jaw pain. Her past medical history was significant for hyperlipidemia and carotid artery

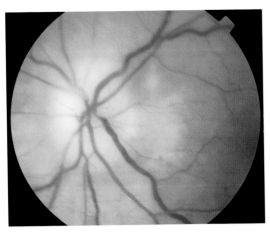

Figure 12.1 Fundus photograph of an 83-year-old, active widow with acute visual loss in the left eye and recent systemic symptoms. The left disc exhibits a distinctive combination of pallor and swelling (pallid edema).

stenosis treated with bilateral carotid endarterectomies 15 years previously. A CBC showed mild normochromic normocytic anemia and Westergren erythrocyte sedimentation rate was 50 mm/hour.

A presumptive diagnosis of anterior ischemic optic neuropathy secondary to giant cell arteritis (GCA) was made. She was given a prescription for oral prednisone 80 mg per day and advised to take calcium supplementation, vitamin D and antacids. A temporal artery biopsy performed two days later was negative, as was a contralateral biopsy performed three days later. Within one week on steroids the patient felt much better and had resumed her usual activities. Her appetite and energy were restored, jaw claudication was gone and her joint stiffness was much improved. She complained, however of "the jitters" and suffered severe insomnia. A repeat ESR was just 4 mm/hour. Because of these steroid side-effects and lack of histopathologic evidence of GCA, she was rapidly weaned off prednisone over the next seven days.

Shortly thereafter, she began to experience episodes of foggy vision in her right eye and mild jaw fatigue when eating. Two days after onset of these symptoms she suddenly lost vision in her right eye while watching television. Examination revealed count fingers vision in her right eye and pallid disc edema. Her prednisone was immediately increased back to 80 mg daily but she never recovered vision in either eye and, due to her severe visual disability, eventually moved into an assisted facility.

The occurrence of bilateral sequential AION in very brief succession, as in this case, is virtually diagnostic of giant cell arteritis. The diagnosis had been suspected on clinical grounds but discarded based on a normal erythrocyte sedimentation rate and bilateral negative temporal artery biopsies. This case raises questions regarding the criteria for making a diagnosis of GCA and some aspects of treatment.

Discussion: There is no blood test that is diagnostic for GCA, but serum markers are routinely used to support a clinical suspicion of the diagnosis. The most commonly employed such test is the erythrocyte sedimentation rate (ESR). Normal values for the ESR increase with age. One commonly used formula defines the normal range as less than age divided by 2 for men and age plus 10 divided by 2 for women. The ESR is elevated in most patients with GCA but 15 to 20% of patients with biopsy-proven GCA have an ESR ≤50 mm/hour. Therefore a normal sedimentation rate does not rule out a diagnosis of GCA. The C-reactive protein (CRP) is a more sensitive serum marker of inflammation, reaching about 98% sensitivity in active GCA. Performing both an ESR and CRP has only a slightly higher yield for detecting an abnormal result than performing a CRP alone. Nonetheless, both laboratory tests should be obtained whenever possible because when both the ESR and CRP are elevated in a patient with clinical features suggestive of GCA the specificity approaches 97%. Conversely, normal values for both tests make a diagnosis of GCA unlikely. Other laboratory findings that are common in GCA are normocytic anemia, leukocytosis and thrombocytosis.

Although histopathologic demonstration of vasculitis by temporal artery biopsy remains the gold standard for the diagnosis of giant cell arteritis, biopsy results, even from an adequate specimen (2 cm or longer), are not always reliable. A negative biopsy result is found in 10–15% of patients in whom the diagnosis is subsequently made on clinical grounds, as in the case above. The additional yield from a second biopsy is low, ranging from 5–9% in different series. Thus, negative temporal artery (TA) biopsy, even when bilateral, does not rule out a diagnosis of GCA. Because biopsy results are occasionally misleading, it is important to be aware of those clinical features that should nevertheless suggest a diagnosis of GCA.

In the setting of acute AION, several clinical features are strongly suggestive of GCA. Age greater than 80 years makes GCA highly likely, as the non-arteritic form rarely affects individuals of advanced age. Other historic features that suggest GCA are: recent headache, jaw claudication, preceding episodes of transient visual loss,

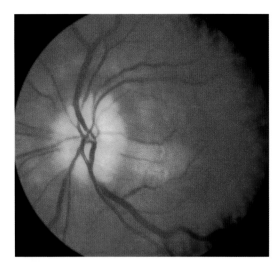

Figure 12.2 Combined disc and retinal edema, due to acute anterior ischemic optic neuropathy and cilioretinal artery occlusion, respectively, in a different patient with GCA.

constitutional symptoms (polymyalgia rheumatica, anorexia, fever) and elevated ESR/CRP. Examination findings that point to the arteritic form of AION include: markedly severe visual loss, pallid disc edema, cotton-wool spots in the retina of either eye, associated cilioretinal artery occlusion and a large cup/disc (C/D) ratio in the contralateral eye (Figures 12.2 and 12.3). These clinical features must all be considered when determining the significance of a negative TA biopsy. For example, an 82-year-old patient with light perception vision due to AION and a generous C/D ratio in the contralateral eye should be assumed to have GCA, regardless of the results of ancillary testing, including TA biopsy.

One important reason for distinguishing arteritic AION from the more common non-arteritic form concerns the visual prognosis for the fellow eye. Among patients with arteritic AION, 25–50%, if untreated, will suffer a similar event in the other eye, usually within 1–14 days. With prompt steroid treatment, such additional visual loss is rare.

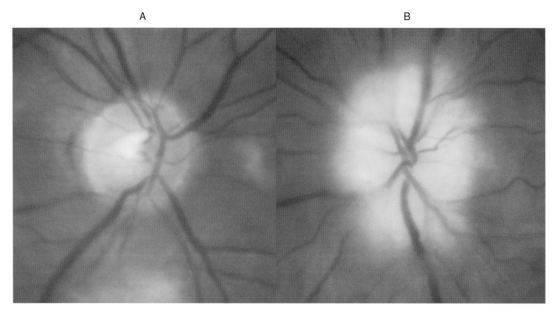

A   B

Figure 12.3 Octogenarian with acute visual loss in the left eye due to arteritic AION. (A) The right disc is flat and has a generous cup/disc ratio. This disc configuration would be highly atypical in a patient with the non-arteritic form of AION. There are also several peri-papillary cotton-wool spots. (B) The left disc shows diffuse pallid swelling.

Treatment of GCA is aimed primarily at preventing ischemic complications such as visual loss, neurologic dysfunction and other organ infarction. Corticosteroids are the mainstay of treatment for this purpose. There is general agreement regarding the need to initiate corticosteroids immediately upon suspicion of GCA, however, the dosage, route of administration, and duration of treatment remain controversial. While there is an abundance of anecdotal evidence regarding treatment, there are no randomized, controlled studies evaluating and comparing the different steroid regimens that are used in the treatment of this disease.

Patients with visual or neurologic symptoms or signs should receive a high initial steroid dose, equivalent to 60 mg or more of prednisone daily. In the setting of transient or acute visual loss, intravenous administration is appropriate, consisting of methylprednisolone 1 gram per day for three to five days. Patients should be hospitalized to monitor for potential adverse reactions including cardiac arrhythmia, acute psychosis, sepsis and anaphylaxis. At discharge they are switched to high dose oral treatment. In patients *without* visual or neurologic manifestations, steroids can be given orally as 60 to 80 mg per day of prednisone (or 1 mg/kg per day). To expedite and ensure prompt treatment, an initial steroid dose can be given before sending the patient home, either as dexamethasone 10 mg IV push or prednisone 80 mg by mouth.

Once treatment is initiated, high dose oral prednisone (60 mg or more) should be maintained for at least four to six weeks, which is generally sufficient time for resolution of systemic symptoms and normalization of serologic markers of disease activity (ESR and/or CRP). Thereafter, steroid tapering is a slow and individualized process. Serologic markers respond more quickly to steroids than do the clinical manifestations of the disease. It is often tempting to stop treatment prematurely in response to adverse side-effects, especially when laboratory tests have returned to normal. This temptation should be resisted. Overall, neuro-ophthalmologists tend to recommend a longer period of high dose prednisone compared to rheumatologists, presum-

ably because of a heightened awareness of cases such as the one described above. As a general rule, the prednisone dose is reduced by 5–10 mg per month, reaching 40 mg daily after two to three months of treatment in most cases. Thereafter, the rate of reduction proceeds more slowly, usually by 5 mg per month. When the daily dose reaches 10–15 mg, tapering may be by as little as 1–2 mg per month. Clinical evaluation and laboratory markers are repeated before each reduction in steroids. Any recurrence of symptoms or rise in ESR or CRP should suggest reactivation of disease activity and should prompt a thorough re-evaluation of treatment. It is important to keep in mind the alternative possibility of a secondary infection in this immunocompromised population. In one study of 145 patients with biopsy-positive GCA, the average time to reach the lowest maintenance dose (median 7 mg daily) was two years. In this study, 92% of patients were still on steroids two years after diagnosis.

Tip: In a patient with suspected giant cell arteritis, certain clinical features should override a negative temporal artery biopsy. Adequate treatment of GCA requires several months of high-dose steroids to adequately suppress active inflammation. Premature tapering of treatment may result in severe visual loss or other ischemic complications.

Overzealous treatment of blood pressure in NAION

Case: A 58-year-old bus driver awoke with decreased vision in the left eye unassociated with head or eye pain, other focal deficits or recent systemic symptoms. His past medical history was positive for systemic hypertension and coronary artery disease. Examination showed visual acuity of 20/20 in each eye with a superior altitudinal defect in the left eye. The right optic disc was flat with no physiologic cup; the left disc was swollen and hyperemic inferiorly.

A diagnosis of non-arteritic anterior ischemic optic neuropathy (NAION) was made and the patient was referred to his primary care physician for further evaluation and treatment. Blood pressure was 140/85 and a general physical examination was unrevealing. Laboratory testing included a CBC, ESR, CRP, fasting blood sugar and lipid profile, all of which were normal. The patient was already on an angiotensin converting enzyme (ACE) inhibitor taken each morning, but in light of his recent vascular event, it was felt that more aggressive blood pressure management would be appropriate. He was therefore told to take a second dose at bedtime and a calcium channel blocker was added.

Two weeks later, vision in the left eye declined further to 20/200 with new appearance of an inferior scotoma. The bottom half of the disc was now pale and the superior portion was swollen.

Discussion: The pathogenesis of NAION is multifactorial, including elements of underlying optic disc structure, atherosclerosis and relative hypotension among other possible factors (see Chapter 11, Acute unilateral visual loss with disc edema). In the management of patients with this common form of optic neuropathy it is important to look for and correct any possible contributory factors. Patients should be specifically questioned regarding recent changes in anti-hypertensive medications, especially nighttime dosing, and the use of other medications that might have a hypotensive or vasoconstrictive effect, such as beta-blockers, diuretics, decongestants, and agents for erectile dysfunction. Efforts should be made to reverse any possible systemic factors that may have played a role in disc infarction. In the case of hypotension this might include discontinuing or decreasing the dose of anti-hypertensive medications or changing the timing of the medication dose. In the setting of acute NAION, it may be appropriate to intentionally allow the blood pressure to drift up a bit until disc edema has subsided. In cases of an acute drop in perfusion pressure, the use of pressor agents, colloid and blood replacement may be considered. This most often occurs in ischemic optic neuropathy associated with dialysis, hemorrhage and certain surgical procedures. In cases with significant anemia or hypoxemia, efforts should be made to correct these factors.

Obstructive sleep apnea syndrome may play a role in some cases of NAION and it is therefore appropriate to inquire about prominent snoring with apneic spells, excessive daytime somnolence and recent weight gain, particularly in portly, middle-aged men.

There is no known effective treatment for NAION. A variety of treatment modalities have been tried, but none with proven efficacy. Corticosteroids and hyperbaric oxygen have not been found to be beneficial. On theoretical grounds, brimonidine may exert a neuroprotective effect at the level of the optic disc and has therefore been advanced as a potential treatment for NAION, but as yet there are no clinical data to demonstrate its efficacy. Initial enthusiasm for optic nerve sheath fenestration was not supported by subsequent studies including a prospective, randomized, multi-center trial in which patients treated surgically actually fared worse in terms of visual outcome as compared to non-operated controls. Another form of surgery, radial optic neurotomy, has been tried in a small number of patients but without proven benefit. Treatment with intra-vitreal triamcinolone or bevacizumab has also been reported but data at this point are quite preliminary.

Because patients who have suffered an episode of NAION are at risk for a similar event in the fellow eye, one aspect of treatment concerns efforts to prevent such a repeat occurrence. To this end, it is appropriate to address vascular risk factors such as hypertension, diabetes, hyperlipidemia, smoking and obesity. As a part of this effort, a more aggressive approach to control of hypertension may be undertaken. While this is well-intentioned, it may be counterproductive. As noted above, relative nocturnal hypotension may play a role in the pathogenesis of NAION. It makes sense that further lowering of blood pressure may have a deleterious effect on a disc that is already swollen and ischemic. Approximately one-third of patients with NAION experience additional loss of vision over days to weeks following the acute event, termed "progressive NAION", and it was this subgroup of patients that was the target of ONSF as a potential treatment. In hopes of preventing such further decline it is wise to avoid any additional drop in blood pressure during this initial vulnerable period. Any recently added anti-hypertensive agents may be discontinued and additional medications should be avoided.

Tip: Systemic hypertension is a risk factor for the development of NAION and should be adequately controlled. Excessive lowering of blood pressure, however, should be avoided.

Prednisone for demyelinating optic neuritis

Case: A 24-year-old secretary experienced darkening of vision in her left eye associated with pain on eye movement and globe tenderness. She was previously healthy with no prior history of neurologic symptoms. Four days after onset, examination showed decreased acuity and color vision in the left eye with a large RAPD. Ophthalmoscopic appearance was normal in both eyes. Retrobulbar optic neuritis was diagnosed and confirmed with MRI that showed hyperintensity within the intraorbital optic nerve on post-contrast images (Figure 12.4). The remainder of the brain was normal, specifically there were no white matter lesions. The patient was treated with a 10-day tapering course of oral

prednisone starting at 60 mg/day. She experienced resolution of pain during the course of treatment and progressive improvement of vision over the next two months. Two months later, however, she experienced similar pain and visual loss affecting the left eye, which was again treated with oral prednisone.

Discussion: The use of steroids for optic neuritis has generated controversy for many years. The original debate concerned the possible effect of corticosteroids on visual outcome. This question was difficult to answer because the natural history of the disorder includes good visual recovery in most cases. The Optic Neuritis Treatment Trial (ONTT), a randomized, prospective, double-blinded multicenter trial, addressed this question in a group of 457 patients with acute optic neuritis who received either oral prednisone alone, intravenous methylprednisolone followed by oral prednisone (1 mg/kg for 11 days) or oral placebo. This important study demonstrated that corticosteroid treatment *does not* influence the visual outcome. While patients who received intravenous steroids did recover more rapidly, their final level of vision (assessed with measurements of acuity, visual field, color vision and contrast sensitivity) was no different from that of patients treated with oral prednisone or placebo.

In addition to visual outcome, the ONTT evaluated the effect of steroids on recurrent episodes

A   B

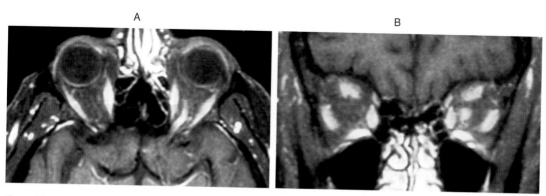

Figure 12.4 Post-contrast fat-suppressed T1-weighted orbital MRI in a 24-year-old secretary with demyelinating optic neuritis. (A) Axial and (B) coronal images show bright enhancement of the posterior portion of the intraorbital left optic nerve.

of demyelination, involving either the optic nerve or the brain. Treatment with intravenous cortico-steroids was associated with half the risk of a repeat demyelinating event over the next two years compared to those who received placebo or oral prednisone. In patients at highest risk for such a repeat event, those with white matter lesions on MRI, the risk decreased from 32% to 16% at two years in the IV steroid-treated group. An unexpected finding in this study was that patients treated with oral prednisone were *twice* as likely to experience recurrent optic neuritis compared to those treated with either IV steroids or placebo. Since the publication of these findings there has been some controversy regarding their significance and validity, including the possibility that what differed between the two steroid-treated groups was not just the route of administration but the dosage. Certainly the dose of steroids used in the intravenous group (250 mg q6h) was significantly higher than that used in the oral prednisone alone group (1 mg/kg per day). This observation has led some clinicians to suggest the use of "megadose" oral steroids, i.e. doses equivalent to those given by IV in the study. Many clinicians have modified the timing of the treatment regimen used in the ONTT, giving the total 1000 mg of methylpred-nisolone as a once-daily infusion instead of the four divided doses used in the study. This modification, coupled with the fact that serious complications of treatment are rare, enables treatment to be given in an outpatient setting. Whether due to the continued debate regarding the scientific basis for the ONTT findings or simply the conservative nature of medical practice, the neurologic community has been relatively slow to adopt the treatment recommendations of the ONTT for the management of acute optic neuritis.

Based on the data from the ONTT, treatment with intravenous steroids should be considered for the following indications: to speed recovery (e.g. for an attack affecting both eyes or an attack in an only good eye) and to decrease the chance of a repeat attack over the next two years in patients at relatively high risk of recurrence (i.e. those with white matter lesions on MRI). Corticosteroid treatment is also appropriate for patients with a known steroid-responsive inflammatory disease (e.g. sarcoidosis or collagen vascular disease). For patients who do not fit any of these indications, the best alternative to IV steroids is *no* treatment, simply reassuring the patient (and oneself) that visual recovery will not be adversely affected by withholding treatment.

Tip: The use of oral corticosteroids should be avoided in patients with acute demyelinating optic neuritis.

Over-reliance on pyridostigmine bromide (Mestinon) in ocular myasthenias

Case: A 75-year-old retired administrator noticed intermittent, painless diplopia two weeks following uncomplicated cataract surgery. Initially, he could force the two images together but now had persistent oblique diplopia in all gaze positions. One week after onset of diplopia, he also developed drooping of the right lid. He was in good general health except for mild hypertension. He had no history of dysphagia, dysarthria, fatigue with chewing or limb weakness.

On examination, there was bilateral ptosis affecting the right eye more than the left with considerable variability and fatigability (Figure 12.5). Adduction and depression of the right eye were limited; eye movements in other directions were full. In primary position there was a large angle exotropia and a right hypertropia. A Tensilon (edrophonium chloride) test was positive, showing complete resolution of ptosis and improvement of eye movements. Further investigation showed no evidence of generalized disease or thymoma.

The patient was started on oral pyridostigmine bromide, starting at 30 mg twice daily with instructions to increase as needed and as tolerated. When he reached 60 mg every six hours he was delighted to find that he no longer had ptosis. The dose was further increased to 90 mg every six hours in an effort to improve his diplopia, but he then developed bouts of explosive diarrhea. He reported that the double images were closer together but he still could not

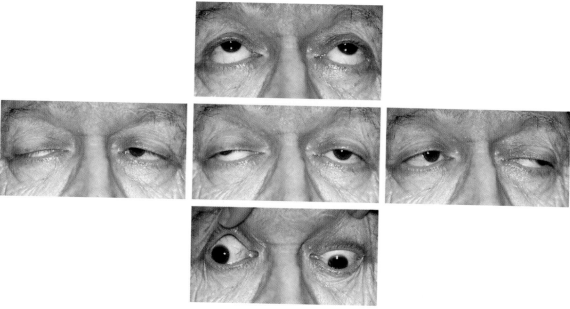

Figure 12.5 Eye movements in a 75-year-old retired administrator with painless diplopia and ptosis. There is marked bilateral ptosis, worse in the right eye, and a large angle right exotropia. In the right eye adduction is mildly limited and depression severely limited. Other eye movements are full.

fuse them into a single image. Variations of the dose and timing of his pyridostigmine bromide were tried over the next six months and an atropinergic agent was added but diarrhea persisted and he began to complain of general lassitude.

In response to his persistent diplopia and adverse side-effects of treatment, pyridostigmine bromide was discontinued and oral prednisone started. After one month he noted resolution of ptosis and dramatic improvement of eye movements. Two months later he was diplopia-free (Figure 12.6).

Discussion: Myasthenia gravis (MG) is caused by auto-antibodies to proteins at the neuromuscular junction. The term "*ocular MG*" (OMG) refers to cases in which disease expression is limited to the extraocular muscles. Patients with OMG seem to have a generally more benign course than those with generalized disease, including a lower risk of malignant thymoma. Nevertheless, OMG can signif-

icantly interfere with activities of daily life and result in significant visual handicap.

There are no large, prospective studies comparing the effectiveness of various treatment modalities for OMG. Treatment options can be divided into supportive measures, acetylcholinesterase inhibitors, and immunosuppressive agents. Supportive and symptomatic treatment measures include lid crutches or tape for ptosis, and prisms or monocular occlusion for diplopia. Prisms have a limited role in the treatment of OMG due to variability in the degree and pattern of misalignment. Surgical procedures (lid or strabismus) are rarely performed and are considered only if the clinical picture has been unchanged for a long period of time.

Acetylcholinesterase (AChE) inhibitors augment the number of available acetylcholine vesicles in the neuromuscular synaptic cleft and are generally considered first line treatment for OMG. Pyridostigmine bromide is the most widely used medication,

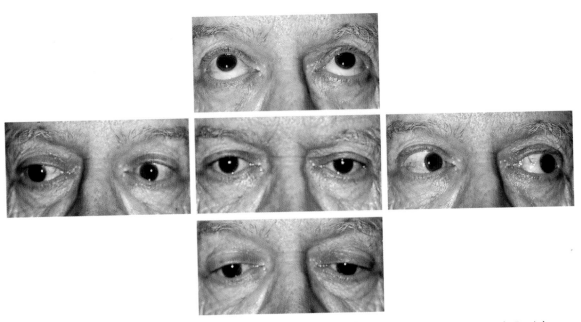

Figure 12.6 Ocular motility in the above patient three months after starting treatment with corticosteroids. Ptosis has resolved, he is aligned in all fields of gaze and eye movements are now completely full.

usually started at 30 mg three times daily and gradually increased to 90–120 mg every four hours. Common side-effects are due to increased muscarinic activity, consisting of abdominal cramps, nausea and diarrhea, which often limit the dose. Side-effects can sometimes be reduced with glycopyrrolate, diphenoxylate and atropine. Bronchospasm and bradycardia can also result and are considered contraindications to the use of this medication.

Although pyridostigmine bromide is a mainstay of treatment for patients with generalized disease, it is not nearly as successful in patients with OMG. The reason for this differential response is unclear. It is possible that extraocular muscles are simply less responsive to AChE inhibitors, or perhaps the metabolic demands of eye muscles are higher than that of other skeletal muscles. Alternatively, the criteria for successful treatment may be more stringent for ocular motility symptoms. If a patient has a weak arm that is 80% better with treatment, he will be pleased with the outcome. But if his eyes are 30 diopters apart and treatment improves them

so that they are now only 5 diopters apart, he will still be diplopic. In addition, ptosis often responds to pyridostigmine bromide more robustly than do the extraocular muscles, and so the patient is more at the mercy of his ocular misalignment because both eyes are now wide open. Whatever the basis for this difference in efficacy, the fact is that only about 10% of patients with diplopia from ocular myasthenia become symptom-free with pyridostigmine bromide. In contrast, most of these patients do extremely well with corticosteroids. The safety profile of pyridostigmine bromide is so favourable compared to that of corticosteroids that an initial trial of an AChE inhibitor is appropriate, but pushing the dose and duration of treatment to the point of unpleasant side-effects without adequate relief of symptoms is not recommended. When starting pyridostigmine bromide for OMG, we would suggest explaining to the patient that there is a good chance this first line of treatment will not be fully effective in relieving diplopia, so as not to lose credibility regarding future treatment options.

The use of steroids in the treatment of OMG remains controversial. While the effectiveness of steroids for preventing progression to generalized MG is unproven, there is no question that most patients with OMG do better symptomatically with prednisone than with pyridostigmine bromide. Corticosteroids achieve improvement of visual symptoms in 70–90% of patients. Outpatient oral therapy is usually employed, starting at low dose and slowly increasing. One suggested protocol consists of prednisone 10 mg every other day, increasing by 10 mg every four days to reach a maximum dose of 80 mg. The dose is then reduced by 10 mg every month down to 30 mg and then by 5 mg each month thereafter. Improvement usually occurs within two weeks of achieving the maximum dose. Long-term, low dose (5 to 10 mg), alternate day treatment is required to maintain remission in about one-third of patients. An alternative approach begins with daily dosing, starting at 10 mg and increasing every three doses to a maximum of 60 mg, then switching to an alternate day regimen once a response has been seen.

While the list of potential complications of steroid treatment is lengthy, the use of alternate day dosing, the relatively short duration of high-dose treatment, and the low dose needed to maintain remission in most patients usually prevent significant long-term adverse effects. The potential for an initial exacerbation of myasthenic weakness upon starting steroid treatment can be prevented by the slow initiation described above. Patients should be monitored for elevations of blood pressure and blood sugar, bone densitometry should be assessed at the onset of treatment, and treatment with a bone sparing agent may be initiated.

For patients who fail to improve with corticosteroids, develop significant steroid side-effects, or cannot reduce their steroid dose below a tolerable amount, other immunosuppressive therapy may be needed. Such modalities include azathioprine, ciclosporin, tacrolimus, mycophenolate mofetil, plasmapheresis and intravenous immunoglobulin (IVIg). Thymectomy has not been widely employed for the management of patients with OMG in the absence of a thymoma. However, as the morbidity of the procedure decreases, particularly via the transcervical route, it is gaining greater acceptance for use in selected patients with OMG.

Until more definitive data are available, management of the patient with OMG must be individualized, specifically balancing the severity of symptoms, the patient's visual requirements and the risk of developing complications of treatment.

Tip: Oral pyridostigmine bromide may improve ptosis, but resolution of diplopia is rarely achieved. Corticosteroids are the mainstay for treatment of ocular myasthenia gravis.

Failure to provide symptomatic treatment

Case: A 62-year-old woman experienced new onset of horizontal diplopia that progressed over one week and then remained stable for the next several months. Her neurologic history was significant for a 30-year history of relapsing remitting multiple sclerosis with secondary progression. She suffered poor balance, moderate spasticity and some loss of sensation in the lower extremities. Examination showed a 35 diopter esotropia with 15 degrees of abduction in the right eye and slowing of right lateral rectus saccades. Her MRI showed extensive white matter disease consistent with demyelinating disease (Figure 12.7). A course of IV methylprednisolone brought no improvement. Initially she wore a patch to prevent diplopia but eventually found that she could ignore one image with both eyes open, but was still troubled by visual confusion and lack of depth perception. Re-evaluation eight months later showed no change. Her deviation was still too large and too incomitant to treat with prisms and she was told that nothing could be done.

She sought a second opinion regarding treatment and, after an additional six month period of observation, was offered the option of strabismus surgery. The potential benefits and risks of surgery were fully discussed, including the possibility that her ocular alignment could change in the future due to progression of her demyelinating disease. She elected to

A   B

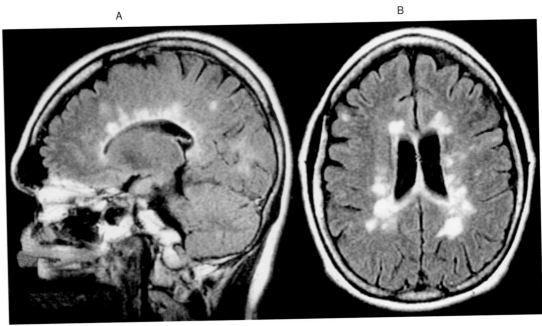

Figure 12.7 FLAIR brain MRI in the above 62-year-old woman with long-standing multiple sclerosis and chronic sixth nerve palsy. (A) Sagittal and (B) axial images show multiple periventricular hyperintensities, including many in the corpus callosum.

undergo extraocular muscle surgery consisting of a recession-resection procedure. Post-operatively her eyes were well aligned in primary position with good range of motion. She remains well four years later.

Discussion: Medical treatment has a range of components. Ideally, we address and correct the underlying disease process and reverse any deficits. In some cases, however, this is not possible and we settle instead for offering prognostic information and comfort. In the face of these limitations we may sometimes neglect forms of treatment that provide only symptomatic relief. In this section, we will address a few examples of such errors of omission.

The ultimate symptomatic treatment for diplopia is occluding one eye (either with a patch or an opaque contact lens) and many patients resort to this option. We can often do better, however. In some cases of ocular misalignment, prisms can restore binocular fusion. In other cases the deviation is too large or too incomitant to treat in this

way and extraocular muscle surgery is needed to re-establish single vision. Even in cases with severe loss of eye muscle function, surgery can often be surprisingly effective. An example of this is the use of full tendon transfer of vertical muscles to restore alignment and some abduction in patients with a complete sixth nerve palsy. Ideally, surgery is postponed until a deficit is stable. However, in some patients whose disorder is expected to be slowly progressive, it may nevertheless be appropriate to intervene surgically at a point when the degree of prism correction becomes cumbersome. The usual limit for ground-in prism is 10 diopters in each lens before spectacles become excessively thick and heavy. Paste-on prisms can be used at higher magnitudes but the resultant blur is often objectionable. Eye muscle surgery can "reset the clock", correcting the motility deficit at least for some period of time. Any subsequent progression can be addressed again with increasing prisms. The above patient is an example of this clinical scenario.

Progressive supranuclear palsy (PSP) is an example of a condition in which there is no effective treatment for the underlying disease process but in which symptomatic measures can be of some benefit. Because PSP usually affects those in mid-life and later, most are wearing bifocals, which do not serve them well as downgaze is progressively limited (see Chapter 9, Chronic progressive external ophthalmoplegia vs. progressive supranuclear palsy). While not a "high-tech" intervention, simply providing separate reading glasses can be extremely helpful for these patients. Because vergence is also impaired, the addition of base-in prism to these reading glasses is often beneficial. An appropriate amount of base-out prism may also be added to distance spectacles to compensate for poor divergence in this condition. Artificial tears can be helpful for the decreased blink rate in PSP as in other parkinsonian syndromes. Providing separate reading glasses is similarly appropriate for any patient with impaired downgaze due to other neurologic disorders.

Most forms of nystagmus and other forms of ocular instability are intractable, but some may show a positive response to medication. Most notably, ocular neuromyotonia typically responds dramatically to carbamazepine and periodic alternating nystagmus often does very well with baclofen. Downbeat nystagmus may dampen with clonazepam but excessive sedation often limits the dose. Certain forms of episodic ataxia with nystagmus respond to acetazolamide. In addition to efforts at pharmacologic treatment, some forms of nystagmus damp with convergence, and in such cases bilateral base-out prism may help stabilize vision by stimulating convergence. In cases with an eccentric null zone (in which nystagmus is absent or decreased with a marked head turn or with chin up or down), bilateral horizontal or vertical prisms or eye muscle surgery can be similarly effective. For intractable cases, botulinum toxin injection into the muscle cone has been used to damp involuntary ocular oscillations by temporarily paralyzing the eye muscles. The downside of such treatment is the resultant loss of the vestibulo-ocular reflex, and the need to patch the fellow eye to avoid diplopia. Large recessions of extraocular muscles have also been employed.

Certain persistent pupillary disorders, while not technically "curable", can be improved with symptomatic measures. The ptosis and miosis of an oculosympathetic palsy (Horner syndrome) can often be reversed with topical application of apraclonidine or dilute phenylephrine. An enlarged pupil that constricts poorly to light may cause photophobia that can be relieved with a contact lens that has a small clear opening. When due to postganglionic parasympathetic denervation (an Adie's tonic pupil) dilute pilocarpine can provide similar symptomatic relief.

FURTHER READING

Idiopathic intracranial hypertension

G. Bynke, G. Zemack, H. Bynke, B. Romner, Ventriculoperitoneal shunting for idiopathic intracranial hypertension. *Neurology*, **63** (2004), 1314–16.

K. B. Digre, J. J. Corbett, Idiopathic intracranial hypertension (pseudotumor cerebri): a reappraisal. *Neurologist*, **7** (2001), 2–67.

H. J. Sugarman, W. F. Felton III, J. B. Salvant Jr., A. Sismanis, J. M. Kellum, Effects of surgically induced weight loss on idiopathic intracranial hypertension in morbid obesity. *Neurology*, **45** (1995), 1655–9.

M. Thambisetty, P. F. Lavin, N. J. Newman, V. Biousse, Fulminant idiopathic intracranial hypertension. *Neurology*, **68** (2007), 229–32.

Giant cell arteritis

S. C. Carroll, B. J. Gaskin, H. V. Danesh-Meyer, Giant cell arteritis. *Clin Exp Ophthalmol*, **334** (2006), 159–73.

J. K. Hall, L. J. Balcer, Giant cell arteritis. *Curr Treat Opt Neurol*, **6** (2004), 45–53.

S. S. Hayreh, B. Zimmerman, Management of giant cell arteritis. *Ophthalmologica*, **217** (2003), 239–59.

Non-arteritic anterior ischemic optic neuropathy

A. C. Arnold, L. A. Levin, Treatment of ischemic optic neuropathy. *Semin Ophthalmol*, **17** (2002), 39–46.

S. Connolly, K. Gordon, J. Horton, Salvage of vision after hypotension-induced ischemic optic neuropathy. *Am J Ophthalmol*, **117** (1994), 235–42.

S. S. Hayreh, B. Zimmerman, P. Podhajsky, W. Alward, Nocturnal arterial hypertension and its role in optic nerve head and ocular ischemic disorders. *Am J Ophthalmol*, **117** (1994), 603–24.

K. Landau, J. M. Winterkorn, L. U. Mailloux, W. Vetter, B. Napolitano, 24-hour blood pressure monitoring in patients with anterior ischemic optic neuropathy. *Arch Ophthalmol*, **114** (1996), 570–5.

The Ischemic Optic Neuropathy Decompression Trial Research Group, Optic nerve decompression surgery for nonarteritic anterior ischemic optic neuropathy (NAION) is not effective and may be harmful. *JAMA*, **273** (1995), 625–32.

Optic neuritis

A. Arnold, Evolving management of optic neuritis and multiple sclerosis. *Am J Ophthalmol*, **139** (2005), 1101–8.

R. W. Beck, P. A. Clear, J. D. Trobe *et al.*, The effect of corticosteroids for acute optic neuritis on the subsequent development of multiple sclerosis. The Optic Neuritis Study Group. *N Engl J Med*, **329** (1993), 1764–9.

S. A. Morrow, C. A. Stoian, J. Dmitrovic, S. C. Chan, L. M. Metz, The bioavailability of IV methylprednisolone and oral prednisone in multiple sclerosis. *Neurology*, **63** (2004), 1079–80.

J. D. Trobe, P. C. Sieving, K. E. Guire, A. M. Fendrick, The impact of the optic neuritis treatment trial on the practices of ophthalmologists and neurologists. *Ophthalmology*, **106** (1999), 2047–53.

Ocular myasthenia

P. S. Chavis, D. E. Stickler, A. Walker, Immunosuppression or surgical treatment for ocular myasthenia gravis. *Arch Neurol*, **64** (2007), 1792–4.

A. Evoli, A. P. Batocchi, C. Minisci, C. DiSchino, P. Tonali, Therapeutic options in ocular myasthenia gravis. *Neuromusc Dis*, **11** (2001), 208–16.

M. E. Gilbert, E. A. DeSousa, P. J. Savino, Ocular myasthenia gravis treatment. The case against prednisone therapy and thymectomy. *Arch Neurol*, **64** (2007), 1790–2.

M. Kupersmith, G. Ying, Ocular motor dysfunction and ptosis in ocular myasthenia gravis: effects of treatment. *Br J Ophthalmol*, **89** (2005), 1330–4.

L. L. Kusner, A. Puwanant, H. Kaminski, Ocular myasthenia. Diagnosis, treatment and pathogenesis. *Neurologist*, **12** (2006), 231–9.

N. T. Monsul, H. S. Patwa, A. M. Knowrr, R. L. Lesser, J. M. Goldstein, The effect of prednisone on the progression from ocular to generalized myasthenia gravis. *J Neurol Sci*, **217** (2004), 131–3.

Nystagmus

R. J. Leigh, R. L. Tomsak, Drug treatments for eye movement disorders. *J Neurol Neurosurg*, **74** (2003), 1–4.

R. McLean, F. Proudlock, S. Thomas, C. Degg, I. Gottlob, Congenital nystagmus: randomized, controlled, double-masked trial of memantine/gabapentin. *Ann Neurol*, **61** (2007), 130–8.

Index